Best Practices for Documenting Occupational Therapy Services in Schools

BEST PRACTICES FOR
Documenting
Occupational Therapy Services
in Schools

Gloria Frolek Clark, PhD, OTR/L, SCSS, BCP, FAOTA, and
Dottie Handley-More, MS, OTR/L

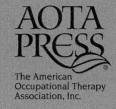

AOTA
PRESS®

The American
Occupational Therapy
Association, Inc.

AOTA *Vision 2025*
Occupational therapy maximizes health, well-being, and quality of life for all people, populations, and communities through effective solutions that facilitate participation in everyday living.

MISSION STATEMENT
The American Occupational Therapy Association advances the quality, availability, use, and support of occupational therapy through standard-setting, advocacy, education, and research on behalf of its members and the public.

AOTA STAFF
Frederick P. Somers | *Executive Director*
Christopher M. Bluhm | *Chief Operating Officer*

Chris Davis | *Director, AOTA Press*
Caroline Polk | *Digital Manager and* AJOT *Managing Editor*
Ashley Hofmann | *Development/Acquisitions Editor*
Barbara Dickson | *Production Editor*

Rebecca Rutberg | *Director, Marketing*
Amanda Goldman | *Marketing Manager*
Jennifer Folden | *Marketing Specialist*

AMERICAN OCCUPATIONAL THERAPY ASSOCIATION, INC.
4720 Montgomery Lane
Bethesda, MD 20814
Phone: 301-652-AOTA (2682)
Fax: 301-652-7711
www.aota.org
To order: 1-877-404-AOTA or store.aota.org

DISCLAIMERS
This publication is designed to provide accurate and authoritative information in regard to the subject matter covered. It is sold or distributed with the understanding that the publisher is not engaged in rendering legal, accounting, or other professional service. If legal advice or other expert assistance is required, the services of a competent professional person should be sought.
—*From the Declaration of Principles jointly adopted by the American Bar Association and a Committee of Publishers and Associations*

It is the objective of the American Occupational Therapy Association to be a forum for free expression and interchange of ideas. The opinions expressed by the contributors to this work are their own and not necessarily those of the American Occupational Therapy Association.

ISBN: 978-1-56900399-2
Library of Congress Control Number: 2017932929

Cover design by Debra Naylor, Naylor Design, Inc., Washington, DC
Composition by Automated Graphics Systems, Inc., White Plains, MD
Printed by Automated Graphics Systems, Inc., White Plains, MD

DEDICATION

We dedicate this to Leslie Jackson and our ASPIIRE Cadre for School Practice who advocated for advancing the role of occupational therapy in schools (our "best buddies" and "mini-me's"); to Sandy Schefkind and the Communities of Practice who have been requesting a book on documentation; to our mentors and colleagues who understand the need for data-based decision making; to the children, families, and educators who are our partners in achieving participation and positive outcomes; and to our own families who support and love us.

CONTENTS

LIST OF FORMS, FIGURES, EXHIBITS, AND TABLES

FORMS

FIGURES

EXHIBITS

TABLES

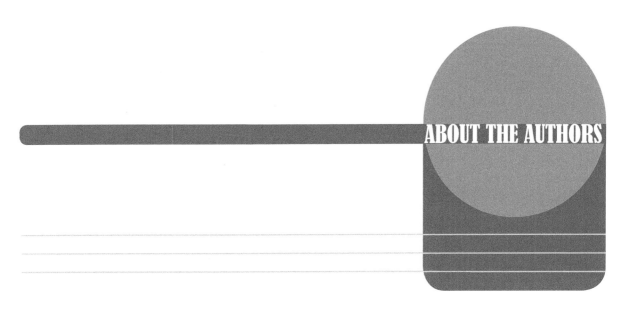

Gloria Frolek Clark, PhD, OTR/L, BCP, SCSS, FAOTA, is a graduate of the University of North Dakota's occupational therapy program. She received her doctorate in Human Development and Family Studies (emphasis on early childhood special education) from Iowa State University in 2010. Dr. Frolek Clark was co-founder of the American Occupational Therapy Association's (AOTA's) Early Intervention and School Special Interest Section (EISSIS) and served on various commissions, including the Commission on Practice (CoP; co-authoring the original *Occupational Therapy Practice Framework*) and Commission on Continuing Competence and Professional Development (serving on Board Certification for Pediatrics and Specialty Certification School System panels).

Dr. Frolek Clark has earned Board Certification in Pediatrics and Specialty Certification in School System, is a Fellow of AOTA, and received AOTA's Recognition of Achievement award. Currently, she is an AOTA Board Director. In 2013, she co-edited the bestselling *Best Practices for Occupational Therapy in Schools* and co-authored *Occupational Therapy Practice Guidelines for Early Childhood: Birth Through Five Years.*

Dr. Frolek Clark has worked in a variety of practice settings (e.g., school, home, community, medical settings, academic) and in policy (Iowa Department of Education). In 2010 she took early retirement from the Iowa Department of Education and works in her private practice. In addition to presentations and publications, she provides consultation for school systems in the United States on program evaluation, provides services to individuals and families, and has taught at

Drake University's occupational therapy doctorate program. Living in Iowa with her husband, she considers herself blessed to have her 3 children's families nearby (including 4 amazing grandchildren).

Dottie Handley-More, MS, OTR/L, is a graduate of the University of Washington's occupational therapy program, where she also received a postprofessional master of science degree in rehabilitation medicine (occupational therapy pathway), specializing in pediatric emotional and behavioral disorders. With over 30 years of experience working in public schools, she has been involved in state and national leadership activities, including serving as chairperson of the EISSIS; Special Interest Section Liaison to the CoP; and co-chairperson of Occupational Therapists in Schools, a special interest section of the Washington Occupational Therapy Association.

Ms. Handley-More has published and presented on a variety of topics related to school-based practice. She was a chapter author for *Best Practices for Occupational Therapy in Schools* and for *Occupational Therapy Services for Children and Youth Under the Individuals with Disabilities Education Act, 3rd Edition.*

Currently, Ms. Handley-More is an occupational therapist and assistive technology consultant for Highline Public Schools and a clinical assistant professor in the Division of Occupational Therapy, Department of Rehabilitation Medicine, at the University of Washington in Seattle, where she lives with her husband, daughter, and 2 cats.

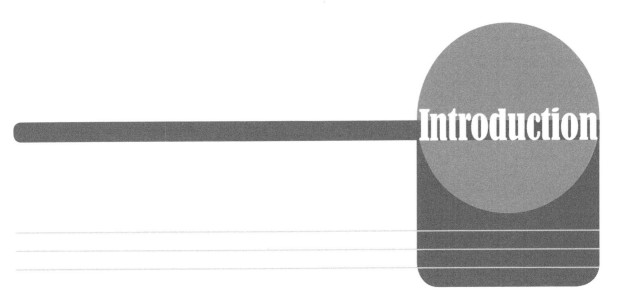

Introduction

OVER THE PAST SEVERAL YEARS, school accountability has become a fundamental aspect of education policy. Amendments to education law mandated rigorous academic standards, measuring student progress against these standards, and establishing consequences for the outcomes (e.g., underachieving schools). Funding for schools is often limited, which means accountability is essential. As service providers in the schools, occupational therapy practitioners are held accountable for their services. Are these services making a difference? Are students who receive occupational therapy services able to benefit from their educational program?

Documentation should provide a trail of data that supports service delivery by occupational therapy practitioners. When documentation provides quantitative data (e.g., student initiated the fine motor classroom activity but could not sustain attention after 2 minutes and needed 5 verbal cues from an adult to complete the task during 10 minutes) instead of qualitative data (e.g., student was unable to finish his fine motor classroom activity), the education team can determine the significance of the problem and monitor change with instruction or intervention. When a student's performance is compared to expectations on the basis of school policy, curricula standards, teacher expectations, or peer performance (e.g., 18 peers in the classroom completed the fine motor activity independently during 10 minutes), discrepancy in a student's performance can be measured for decision making.

Simple but effective documentation that allows efficient use of the occupational therapist's professional judgement and time is critical. We strived to develop a book that provided forms that allow practitioners to efficiently gather data so you could use professional judgement.

We have organized this book to align with the occupational therapy process. Data collection is first because it provides a foundation for all other areas, from screening and evaluation to intervention, outcomes, program evaluation, and supervision of occupational therapy assistants. Each chapter discusses essential considerations regarding relevant federal laws and professional standards and provides strategies for efficiently documenting occupational therapy services.

We admit to a passion for data collection and forms! When others ask "how can we do that?" we are the ones scribbling and drawing a new form on paper, or arranging columns and rows in our heads for new forms. Writing this book and developing new forms has been fun and, we are glad to share dozens of forms with you. These forms are intended as examples that you can use and integrate into your setting. Although these forms are copyrighted, they may be freely used by practitioners in schools for documentation purposes. The flash drive accompanying this text includes fillable forms that may be printed or saved electronically.

We hope that when you open this book, it will spark your own ideas of how you can collect and display data for decision making about service needs and effectiveness. We hope you are inspired to create forms to meet the unique needs within your setting. Finally, we hope that you too will get hooked on data and documentation.

—Gloria & Dottie

Introduction to Documentation in Schools

Documentation is a process of recording professional services provided by occupational therapy practitioners within their scope of practice (American Occupational Therapy Association [AOTA], 2013). Its purpose is to communicate information about a client, articulate the rationale for providing occupational therapy services, and create a chronological record of the depth and breadth of services (AOTA, 2013).

During service provision in preschools and schools, occupational therapy practitioners[1] gather data—typically, qualitative and quantitative data—from multiple sources for decision making, establishing goals, monitoring progress, and promoting effective outcomes for children and youth (Frolek Clark, Cahill, & Ivey, 2015). These data and services are documented according to state licensure as well as professional standards and ethics. Occupational therapy practitioners must follow the minimum standard of documentation established by AOTA and published as standards of practice and guidelines (AOTA, 2013, 2014a, 2014b, 2015a, 2015b). (*Note.* AOTA's *Guidelines for Documentation of Occupational Therapy* is available in Appendix A, and *Standards of Practice for Occupational Therapy* is available in Appendix B.)

---

[1]*Occupational therapy practitioners* refers to occupational therapists and occupational therapy assistants.

TABLE 1.1.   FEDERAL, STATE, AND LOCAL LAWS AND PROCEDURES REQUIRING DOCUMENTATION

FEDERAL	STATE	LOCAL
Individuals With Disabilities Education Improvement Act of 2004 Every Student Succeeds Act of 2015 Family Educational Rights and Privacy Act of 1974 Improving Head Start for School Readiness Act of 2007 Healthy Hunger-Free Kids Act of 2010 (National School Breakfast and Lunch program) Health Insurance Portability and Accountability Act of 1996 Section 504 of the Rehabilitation Act of 1973, as amended Social Security Act of 1965 (Medicaid)	Professional regulatory law (i.e., licensure) Department of Education administrative rules Department of Education special education law Medicaid state programs	School district policies and procedures Policies and procedures of any LEAs that provide services to school districts

Note. LEAs = local education agencies.

LEGAL REQUIREMENTS

Occupational therapy practitioners are responsible for understanding and providing services that adhere to federal laws as well as the rules and policies of state education agencies (SEAs), local education agencies (LEAs), and school districts. Most of these laws and local policies and procedures require documentation (see Table 1.1). In general, the school district, state department of education, or school agency has developed a set of standard forms to meet the requirements of federal and state laws (e.g., individualized education programs [IEPs], authorization for release of information, consent for services; see Table 1.2 for federal laws and regulations). Forms specific for occupational therapy services are generally the responsibility of the occupational therapy practitioners working in that district or agency. To develop these forms, practitioners working in educational settings must be aware of requirements established by their state regulatory board (licensure) and state laws as well as professional standards established by AOTA (see Table 1.1).

This book is designed to assist occupational therapy practitioners in accessing forms that are efficient and simple to use. To accommodate the preference of various users, some forms are presented in multiple formats and with some examples.

TABLE 1.2.   EXAMPLES OF PROFESSIONAL AND FEDERAL DOCUMENTATION REQUIREMENTS FOR OCCUPATIONAL THERAPY PRACTITIONERS WORKING IN SCHOOLS

PROCESS AREA OF OCCUPATIONAL THERAPY SERVICE DELIVERY	AOTA DOCUMENTS (ALSO CONSIDER YOUR STATE'S REGULATORY LAWS)	FEDERAL LAWS AND REGULATIONS (ALSO CONSIDER YOUR STATE'S EDUCATION LAWS)
Overview	*Framework:* "Achieving health, well-being, and participation in life through engagement in occupation" (AOTA, 2014b, p. S2). *Standards of Practice for Occupational Therapy:* Educates referral sources about the scope of occupational therapy services and referral process (AOTA, 2015b). *Occupational Therapy Code of Ethics:* Practitioners must demonstrate concern for the safety and well-being of the client; refrain from actions that cause harm; respect rights of the person to self-determination, privacy, confidentiality, and consent; promote fairness and objectivity during service delivery; provide comprehensive, accurate, and objective information about occupational therapy; and treat clients, colleagues, and other professionals with respect, discretion, fairness, and integrity (AOTA, 2015a).	Specialized instructional support personnel, which includes occupational therapy, can provide consultation for, and participate in, school-wide programs to improve student performance (ESSA). "Related services . . . as may be required to assist a child with a disability to benefit from special education" (IDEA, §1401[26][A]). *Note.* Some states allow occupational therapy to be a support service, meaning occupational therapy may be the only special education service on a child's IEP. FERPA and HIPAA require confidentiality of all verbal, written, electronic, and nonverbal communications relating to a student.

(Continued)

TABLE 1.2. EXAMPLES OF PROFESSIONAL AND FEDERAL DOCUMENTATION REQUIREMENTS FOR OCCUPATIONAL THERAPY PRACTITIONERS WORKING IN SCHOOLS *(CONT.)*

PROCESS AREA OF OCCUPATIONAL THERAPY SERVICE DELIVERY	AOTA DOCUMENTS (ALSO CONSIDER YOUR STATE'S REGULATORY LAWS)	FEDERAL LAWS AND REGULATIONS (ALSO CONSIDER YOUR STATE'S EDUCATION LAWS)
Domain and disability categories	Occupational therapy practitioners work with students who have various physical, mental health, and intellectual disabilities. *Framework:* Domain—occupations,[a] client factors,[b] performance skills,[c] performance patterns,[d] context,[e] and environment.[f]	*Educational disabilities in IDEA:* Intellectual disabilities, hearing impairments (including deafness), speech or language impairments, visual impairments (including blindness), serious emotional disturbance (emotional disturbance), orthopedic impairments, autism, traumatic brain injury, other health impairments, or specific learning disability (§1401[3][A][i]).
Screening	*Standards of Practice for Occupational Therapy:* Obtain and review data to determine the need for further evaluation and intervention; the OT communicates screening results and recommendations to appropriate person, group, or organization. *Guidelines for Documentation of Occupational Therapy:* Document referral source, reason for screening, and need for evaluation and service; includes brief assessment to determine client's need for occupational therapy evaluation or for referral to another service; suggested content provided in original document. *OTA supervision:* The OT is responsible for service delivery and delegating responsibilities. This includes determining the need for services and complexity of the client's needs and condition (AOTA, 2014a).	*IDEA mentions screening in relation to early intervening services:* Rule of construction allows screening to determine appropriate instructional strategies for curriculum implementation; this shall not be considered an evaluation for eligibility for special education and related services (§1414[a][1][E]). IDEA states that children with disabilities must be identified under Child Find: Identify, locate, and evaluate children with disabilities who need special education and related services (§300.111[a][1]). Note different purposes: *General education*—Identify instructional strategies for the classroom. *Special education*—Determine whether the child has a disability that requires special education and related services.
Evaluation		
Evaluation	*Standards of Practice for Occupational Therapy:* Collaboratively with the client, the OT evaluates the client's ability to participate in daily life tasks, roles, and responsibilities and considers the client's history, goals, and needs, as well as the activities and occupations the client wants or needs to complete within the environments and context. The OT obtains and interprets data, plans the intervention, and documents the evaluation process and results. *Framework:* Completing the Occupational Profile assists the OT in understanding the client's history and experience as well as his or her reasons for seeking services and strengths and concerns in occupations (daily life activities). The Occupational Profile considers context or environment, client factors, activity demands, performance skills, and performance patterns. *Guidelines for Documentation of Occupational Therapy:* The OT documents client information and diagnosis, referral information, occupational profile, assessments used and results, and analysis of occupational performance and provides a summary based on initial concern and recommendations regarding need for occupational therapy services. *OTA supervision* (i.e., *Guidelines for Supervision, Roles, and Responsibilities During the Delivery of Occupational Therapy Services;* AOTA, 2014a): The OT is responsible for service delivery and delegating responsibilities. The OTA contributes to the process.	Full and individual initial evaluation requires parent consent and is used to determine whether the child has a disability and is eligible for special education and related services (IDEA, §1414[a][1]). Initial evaluation must be completed within 60 days of receiving parental consent for evaluation. Procedures must determine whether this child has a disability and his or her educational needs (IDEA, §300.301). A copy of the evaluation report must be provided to the parents at no cost (IDEA, §300.306). *Evaluation:* The OT, agency, or school district shall provide notice to the parents and describe any evaluation procedure the agency proposes to conduct (IDEA, §1414[b] and [c]). A variety of assessment tools and strategies are used to gather relevant functional, developmental, and academic information about the child, including information from the parent. Information should directly assist in determining the educational needs of the child. Content of the IEP includes information about the child's involvement in general education curriculum (or a preschooler's ability to participate in appropriate activities; IDEA, §300.304). As appropriate, existing evaluation data should be reviewed, including information provided by the parent; classroom-based, local, or state assessments; classroom-based observations; and observations by teachers and related service providers. The team must determine whether child has a disability and subsequent educational needs, the present levels of academic achievement and related developmental needs, whether special education and related services are needed, and any additions or modifications to the special education and related services that are needed to meet the child's measurable annual goals (IDEA, §300.305). *Observation:* The child should be observed in his or her learning environment to document academic performance and behaviors in the areas of difficulty (IDEA, §300.310).

(Continued)

TABLE 1.2.   EXAMPLES OF PROFESSIONAL AND FEDERAL DOCUMENTATION REQUIREMENTS FOR OCCUPATIONAL THERAPY PRACTITIONERS WORKING IN SCHOOLS *(CONT.)*

PROCESS AREA OF OCCUPATIONAL THERAPY SERVICE DELIVERY	AOTA DOCUMENTS (ALSO CONSIDER YOUR STATE'S REGULATORY LAWS)	FEDERAL LAWS AND REGULATIONS (ALSO CONSIDER YOUR STATE'S EDUCATION LAWS)
Eligibility	*Standards of Practice for Occupational Therapy:* OTs use current assessments and procedures during screening, evaluation, and reevaluation process and communicates the results. *OTA supervision:* The OT interprets the gathered information and integrates the data into the decision-making process. The OTA contributes by gathering data (e.g., assessments, observations) as delegated by the OT.	*Determine eligibility:* Eligibility under IDEA requires that the child has one of the disabilities identified under IDEA and needs special education and related services[g] (§300.8). After the full and individual initial evaluation (at no cost to the parent), the qualified professionals and the parents determine whether the child has a disability and is eligible for SE and related services. Parents must receive a copy of the evaluation report and documentation of determination of eligibility. A child is not considered to be a child in need if appropriate instruction was not provided; he or she has limited English proficiency; and he or she does not meet eligibility criteria from above (IDEA, §300.306). *Specific documentation for eligibility:* When a child is suspected of having a learning disability, documentation must include relevant behavior; educationally relevant medical findings; whether the child met grade-level standards; and whether the child participated in response to scientific, research-based intervention. The strategies used and data collected must be documented and parents must be provided with documentation about the state's policies regarding this process (IDEA, §300.311).

Intervention

Intervention plan	*Standards of Practice for Occupational Therapy:* The OT completes the intervention plan within the required timeline; collaborates with clients to develop and implement the intervention plan; modifies the intervention plan throughout the intervention; and documents services provided within the time frames, formats, and standards established. *Guidelines for the Documentation of Occupational Therapy:* Intervention plan—On the basis of the results of the evaluation or reevaluation, the OT must document occupational therapy intervention goals, intervention approaches, and types of interventions that will be used to achieve the client's outcomes. Recommendations or referrals to other professionals and agencies are included (AOTA, 2013).[h] *OTA supervision:* The development of the intervention plan is the overall responsibility of the OT, in collaboration with the client and OTA.	*Excusal form:* A member of the IEP team may be excused from attending the IEP meeting if the parents and LEA consent to the excusal and the member submits in writing input to the IEP before the meeting (IDEA, §1414[d][C][ii]). *IEP development:* The IEP team members shall consider the strengths of the child; concerns of the parents for enhancing the child's education; results of the initial evaluation or other evaluations of the child; and the academic, developmental, and functional needs of the child. The IEP must include a written statement of the child's present levels of academic achievement and functional performance, annual goals, and description of progress toward annual goals; statement of special education and related services and supplementary aids and services provided to the child or on behalf of the child; a statement of program modifications or supports for school personnel; a statement about the extent to which the child will not participate with nondisabled children in regular class and activities; a statement of individual appropriate accommodations necessary for state and districtwide assessment; the projected date for beginning of services and anticipated frequency, location, and duration; and a transition IEP when child is 16 years (or according to state education law). This must be updated at least annually (IDEA, §1414[d]).

(Continued)

TABLE 1.2. EXAMPLES OF PROFESSIONAL AND FEDERAL DOCUMENTATION REQUIREMENTS FOR OCCUPATIONAL THERAPY PRACTITIONERS WORKING IN SCHOOLS *(CONT.)*

PROCESS AREA OF OCCUPATIONAL THERAPY SERVICE DELIVERY	AOTA DOCUMENTS (ALSO CONSIDER YOUR STATE'S REGULATORY LAWS)	FEDERAL LAWS AND REGULATIONS (ALSO CONSIDER YOUR STATE'S EDUCATION LAWS)
Intervention implementation	*Standards of Practice for Occupational Therapy:* Use professional and clinical reasoning, evidence-based practice, and therapeutic use of self to implement the most appropriate types of interventions. *Framework:* Types of intervention may include occupations and activities, preparatory methods and tasks, education and training, advocacy, and group interventions. *Guidelines for Documentation of Occupational Therapy:* Summarize the intervention process and document the client's progress toward achievement of goals. Includes new data collected; modifications of treatment plan; and statement of need for continuation, discontinuation, or referral.	*IEP:* The IEP team identifies the special education and related services and supplementary aids and services, based on peer-reviewed research to the extent practicable, to be provided to the child or on behalf of the child; the IEP includes a list of program modifications for school personnel. The team determines the date for beginning services and the anticipated frequency, location, and duration of these services (IDEA, §1414[d]).
Intervention review	*Standards of Practice for Occupational Therapy:* The OT modifies the intervention plan throughout the intervention. *Guidelines for Documentation of Occupational Therapy:* Reevaluation same as for evaluation, with an update on progress included and recommendations with regard to changes to occupational therapy services; revision or continuation of interventions, goals, and objectives; frequency of occupational therapy services; and recommendation for referral to other professionals or agencies as applicable.	*Progress reports:* Progress on annual goals must be measured and reported to parents, concurrent with issuance of report cards (IDEA, §1414[d][1][A][IV]).
Outcomes	*Standards of Practice for Occupational Therapy:* "An [OT] is responsible for documenting changes in the client's performance and capacities and for transitioning the client to other types or intensity of services or discontinuing services when a client has achieved identified goals, reached maximum benefit, or does not desire to continue services" (AOTA, 2015b, p5). An OTA may contribute to the transition plan or the discontinuation plan. *Framework:* Included throughout the occupational therapy service delivery process, outcomes describe the benefit of occupational therapy and are directly connected to the interventions provided. *Guidelines for Documentation of Occupational Therapy:* Discharge report contains a summary of occupational therapy services provided and client outcomes. *Suggested content*—Client information, summary of intervention process from initial evaluation to discontinuation of services, and recommendations for client's future needs.	*Amendments to IEP:* Changes to the IEP may be made by the entire IEP team or by amending the IEP (§1414[d][3][F]). *Review and revision of the IEP:* The child's IEP should be reviewed not less than annually to determine whether the goals are being achieved, and revised as needed (IDEA, §414[d][4]). *Change in eligibility or termination of services:* An evaluation must occur before determining the child no longer has a disability unless the child's services are being terminated because of graduation with a regular diploma or exceeding the age of eligibility under state law (IDEA, §1414[c][5]). *Discontinuation of occupational therapy (related services):* Based on a current reevaluation by the OT, a proposed action of discontinuing occupational therapy is made by the OT to the IEP Team. The parent is provided with a prior written notice that explains the proposed action and a copy of their procedural safeguards (§1415[c][1][B]). *Note.* Collaboration with other members of the IEP team (e.g., family, student, teachers) should occur throughout this process. Input from the team should be solicited prior to an IEP team meeting and especially before any suggestion to discontinue services or change the amount of therapy intervention is presented.

(Continued)

TABLE 1.2 EXAMPLES OF PROFESSIONAL AND FEDERAL DOCUMENTATION REQUIREMENTS FOR OCCUPATIONAL THERAPY PRACTITIONERS WORKING IN SCHOOLS *(CONT.)*

PROCESS AREA OF OCCUPATIONAL THERAPY SERVICE DELIVERY	AOTA DOCUMENTS (ALSO CONSIDER YOUR STATE'S REGULATORY LAWS)	FEDERAL LAWS AND REGULATIONS (ALSO CONSIDER YOUR STATE'S EDUCATION LAWS)
Reevaluation	*Standards of Practice for Occupational Therapy* and *Framework:* Reviews client performance and goals to identify change during intervention (type and amount of change). *Framework:* See "Evaluation" section of table. *Guidelines for Documentation of Occupational Therapy:* Conducts reevaluation on the basis of needs of setting, progress of client, and client changes. Documents results of reevaluation process (see "Evaluation" section). *OTA supervision:* The OT is responsible for service delivery and delegating responsibilities. The OTA contributes to the process.	*Reevaluations:* Reevaluations shall not occur more than once a year unless the parent and public agency agree and must occur at least once every 3 years unless the parent and public agency agree it is not necessary. The parent, public agency, or teacher may determine whether educational or related services indicate reevaluation is necessary (IDEA, §300.303). In addition, determination should be made regarding whether the child continues to have a disability and the educational needs of the child as well as whether special education and related services are necessary (IDEA, §300.305). *Note.* Best practice indicates systematic and frequent data collection to determine the child's progress toward IEP goals.
Payment	*Standards of Practice for Occupational Therapy:* The OT documents therapy provided within the standards, time frames, and formats established by agencies in the practice setting, federal and state laws, other regulatory and payer requirements, and AOTA documents. *OTA supervision:* Must meet regulatory requirements. *Occupational Therapy Code of Ethics:* Refer to "Overview" section of this table. "Terminate occupational therapy services . . . when the services are no longer beneficial" (p. 3); "Report to appropriate authorities any acts in practice . . . that are unethical or illegal" (p. 5); "Ensure that documentation for reimbursement purposes is done in accordance with applicable laws, guidelines, and regulations" (p. 6); "Refrain from using or participating in the use of any form of communication that contains false, fraudulent, deceptive, misleading, or unfair statements or claims" (p. 6).	Medical services provided under the Medicaid program, such as occupational therapy, may be covered for children under IDEA and Section 504. *Extended school year services:* On the basis of the IEP team planning process, services may be provided beyond the typical school year. Occupational therapy services included in an IEP may be covered under the following conditions: services are medically necessary; federal and state Medicaid regulations are followed; and services are included in the state's plan or under Early and Periodic, Screening, Diagnostic and Treatment (CMS, 2003). Practitioners must understand and comply with their state and school district documentation requirements.

Note. AOTA = American Occupational Therapy Association; CMS = Centers for Medicare and Medicaid Services; ESSA = Every Student Succeeds Act of 2015; IDEA = Individuals with Disabilities Education Improvement Act of 2004; IEP = individualized education program; *Framework* = *Occupational Therapy Practice Framework: Domain and Process* (3rd ed., AOTA, 2014b); FERPA = Family Educational Rights and Privacy Act of 1974; HIPAA = Health Insurance Portability and Accountability Act of 1996; LEA = local education agency; OT = occupational therapist; OTA = occupational therapy assistant.

[a]*Occupations* include activities of daily living, instrumental activities of daily living, rest and sleep, education, work, play, leisure, and social participation. [b]*Client factors* include values, beliefs, and spirituality; body functions; and body structures. [c]*Performance skills* include motor skills, process skills, and social interaction skills. [d]*Performance patterns* include person and group. [e]*Context* includes cultural, personal, temporal, and virtual. [f]*Environments* include physical and social. [g]If a student meets the definition of disability but does not require special education, a Section 504 Plan may be necessary. [h]The intervention goals listed above are specific to occupational therapy practice and not the IEP. For example, the IEP team may develop a goal of dressing independently. The OT's intervention may be to enhance finger dexterity so the student can fasten buttons and increase range of motion so the student can reach around and grasp a sleeve.

TECHNOLOGY

Technology offers a variety tools that streamline the documentation process. Although creating a customized form may initially require a significant investment in time, having the right form often saves time in the long run. Common software programs used to create forms include word processing programs and spreadsheet programs. Word processing programs allow the user to type, edit, organize, and format text and insert graphics. There are several common word processing features that can be used to create efficient and effective forms. These features include tables, templates, form fields, and mail merge. Tables organize information into columns and rows. Templates, created from a word processing document such as an outline for an evaluation report, ensure that the original template remains unchanged and cannot be edited accidentally.

Occupational therapists with experience creating word processing or PDF documents may save time by adding form fields within their documents to create fillable forms that can be completed by hand or electronically. Examples of form fields include text boxes, check boxes, and dropdown lists. Mail merge is a feature that allows the user to create a form (e.g., a letter that goes home to parents every year) by entering placeholders for specific information (e.g., a student's first name, last name, and IEP due date). The form is connected to a data source (usually a separate table or spreadsheet document), and data from the source document are matched to the placeholders within the form. Table 1.3 provides an overview of word processing features along with examples of ways in which they can be used.

Similar to tables, spreadsheets sort data into rows and columns. However, spreadsheets offer the option to enter formulas that calculate and analyze the data and use the data to create charts and graphs. For example, an occupational therapy department could enter therapist caseload data into a spreadsheet and add formulas to have the spreadsheet calculate how many preschool, elementary, middle school, and high school students are served by the department each year. The spreadsheet could then create a pie chart to show the percentage of students the department serves at each grade band, and trends could be tracked over time. Table 1.4 provides an overview of common spreadsheet features along with examples of ways in which they can be used.

Web-based technology is another tool school teams are using to streamline the documentation process. This type of technology allows files and folders to be created online or uploaded and saved to a cloud server where they are accessed via the Internet. One of the advantages of using web-based technology is that it allows team members to share documentation forms and fill them out electronically using their mobile devices (e.g., smart phones, tablets, netbooks). For example, an IEP team could create a data collection form for an IEP goal, and multiple team members could access the form and use it to collect data.

Some Internet services provide the option to create fillable forms that automatically send the entered data to a spreadsheet. However, web-based technology may not provide adequate security for confidential information. Teams that use the Internet to share documents and collect data should be careful to maintain student confidentiality by coding student names, avoiding the use of other identifiable

TABLE 1.3.   WORD PROCESSING FEATURES AND EXAMPLES OF USE

FEATURE	ADVANTAGES AND SPECIAL FEATURES	EXAMPLES
Table	• Accommodates large amounts of text and multiple paragraphs • Allows text to be formatted within the cells (e.g., bulleted or numbered lists, indented paragraphs)	• Column-style narrative notes • Checklists and rubrics • Flow sheets
Template	• Automatically creates a new document when opened • Requires user to name the document when saving to prevent changes to the original template	• Evaluation report • Progress report • Intervention plan
Form fields	• Provides a form with blank spaces to fill in and protected areas that cannot be changed • Allows text to be entered or can be formatted to offer choices from a drop-down menu or checklist	• Intervention plans • Referral forms
Mail merge	• Retrieves data from a spreadsheet or table and merges it into a form • Is great for adding student information when the same form is used for many students	• Attendance forms • Therapy log forms that will be filled out by hand

TABLE 1.4. SPREADSHEET FEATURES AND EXAMPLES OF USE

FEATURE	ADVANTAGES AND SPECIAL FEATURES	EXAMPLES
Formulas	• Can count and graph numerical data • Can calculate date and time • Includes multiple mathematical and statistical formulas available	*Note.* Both formulas and data tools could be useful for these forms. • Data collection forms • Time sample data • Progress-monitoring data • Schedule or schedule matrix • Therapy log forms for therapy groups • Task analysis • Caseload lists
Data tools	• Includes fill options and drop-down menus to support data entry • Can group, sort, and filter data • Can be used to insert data into 1 cell, which can then appear in multiple cells on 1 worksheet or multiple worksheets	
Charts and graphs	• Creates a graphic representation using data from a spreadsheet • Offers a variety of graphic options such as pie charts, line graphs, bar graphs, and scatter plots	• Progress reporting chart • Time use data chart

information, and adhering to district policies regarding confidential information.

SUMMARY

Documentation of occupational therapy services in schools must adhere to multiple laws and regulations, including professional requirements. Understanding and following these requirements during service delivery are the responsibility of each occupational therapy practitioner. Using forms that offer efficient ways to record information about the client and services provided is recommended.

REFERENCES

American Occupational Therapy Association. (2013). Guidelines for documentation of occupational therapy. *American Journal of Occupational Therapy, 67*(Suppl.), S32–S38. http://dx.doi.org/10.5014/ajot.62.6.684

American Occupational Therapy Association. (2014a). Guidelines for supervision, roles, and responsibilities during the delivery of occupational therapy services. *American Journal of Occupational Therapy, 68*(Suppl. 3), S16–22. http://dx.doi.org/10.5014/ajot.63.6.797

American Occupational Therapy Association. (2014b). Occupational therapy practice framework: Domain and process (3rd ed.). *American Journal of Occupational Therapy, 68*(Suppl. 1), S1–S48. http://dx.doi.org/10.5014/ajot.2014.682006

American Occupational Therapy Association. (2015a). Occupational therapy code of ethics. *American Journal of Occupational Therapy, 69*(Suppl. 3), 1–8. http://dx.doi.org/10.5014/ajot.2015.696S03

American Occupational Therapy Association. (2015b). Standards of practice for occupational therapy. *American Journal of Occupational Therapy, 69*(Suppl. 3), 1–6. http://dx.doi.org/10.5014/ajot.2015.696S06.

Centers for Medicare and Medicaid Services. (2003). *Medicaid school-based administrative claiming guide.* Retrieved from https://www.cms.gov/research-statistics-data-and-systems/computer-data-and-systems/medicaidbudget expendsystem/downloads/schoolhealthsvcs.pdf

Every Student Succeeds Act of 2015, Pub. L. 114–95 § 114 Stat. 1177 (2015–2016).

Family Educational Rights and Privacy Act of 1974, Pub. L. 93–380, 20 U.S.C. § 1232g, 34 CFR Part 99 et seq.

Frolek Clark, G., Cahill, S., & Ivey, C. (2015). School practice documentation: Documenting and organizing quantitative data. *OT Practice, 20*(15), 12–15.

Health Insurance Portability and Accountability Act of 1996, Pub. L. 104–191 42 U.S.C. § 300gg, 29 U.S.C § 1181-1183, and 42 U.S.C. 1320d-1320d9.

Healthy Hunger-Free Kids Act of 2010, Pub. L. 111–296, CFR Parts 245, 272.

Improving Head Start for School Readiness Act of 2007, Pub. L. 110–134, 121 Stat. 1363.

Individuals With Disabilities Education Improvement Act of 2004, Pub L. 108–446, 20 U.S.C. § § 1400-1482.

Section 504 of the Rehabilitation Act of 1973, Pub. L. 93–112, as amended 29 U.S.C. § 1794 (2008).

Social Security Amendments of 1965, Pub. L. 89–97, 79 Stat. 286, Title XIX.

Data Collection

During service delivery, occupational therapy practitioners gather data to guide decision making about the need for occupational therapy services, the effectiveness of interventions, the need for ongoing services, the need for extended year services, and more. Data-based decision making uses data collected about the student's performance to enhance problem-solving collaboration and demonstrate effectiveness in occupational therapy interventions (Frolek Clark, 2013b; Frolek Clark & Miller, 1996; Handley-More & Chandler, 2008; Linder & Clark, 2000). In this section we explore the use of quantitative data for data collection using progress monitoring, goal attainment scaling, and rubrics.

The purpose and type of data being collected should be based on rigor of the decisions being made. For instance, screening data must identify whether there are areas of risk that require additional assessment, whereas data collected during an evaluation must be more rigorous because they are used to identify discrepancies in activities and occupations the person can and cannot perform (Frolek Clark, 2010; see also Chapter 3, "Tiered Support: Screening and Evaluation," for more information about screening). Data collected for program evaluation must enable decisions to be made about the effectiveness of the program (see Chapter 5, "Outcomes and Program Evaluation," for more information about program effectiveness).

QUALITATIVE VS. QUANTITATIVE DATA

Whereas qualitative data provide information about a student (e.g., "Liam is the last student to dress for recess and has difficulty interacting with other students during recess"), quantitative data provide more specific information needed for intervention planning, especially when a student is being compared with other peers (e.g., peers are dressed for recess in 3 min, whereas Liam requires 7 min and 2 redirectives from an adult. During recess, Liam initiated 0 interactions with peers and responded 20% of the time [1:5] to peer-initiated interactions. Peers made 8 interactions and responded 80% of the time [4:5] to peer-initiated interactions. During the past 2 recesses, Liam sat on the swing for 17 of 20 min. Peers varied their activities on the playground [e.g., ball, swing, climbing toys, tag/running games]).

DATA COLLECTION PROCESS: PROGRESS MONITORING

When collecting data to monitor progress, certain steps should be followed (see Form 2.A, "Steps in Progress Monitoring"). *Progress monitoring* is a scientifically based practice to assess student performance on a regular basis and can be used to identify students in general education who are at risk (e.g., response to intervention, multitiered systems of support) and to determine student performance and rate of progress with supplemental or intensive interventions. When a student is receiving occupational therapy services on an individualized education program (IEP), goals may be monitored using the data collection process to identify the student's progress and the effectiveness of the intervention. Progress monitoring involves these six steps:

1. Define the concern.
2. Select the measurement strategy.
3. Determine the current level of performance (i.e., baseline).
4. Set the goal.
5. Set up a chart.
6. Develop a decision-making plan for use during service provision.

STEP 1. DEFINE THE CONCERN

Beginning the process with the occupational profile allows the occupational therapy practitioner to understand the student's health, developmental history, educational history, and experiences. The values and needs of the educational program and the family also emerge during interviews. Understanding the physical and social environments and activities that are supportive of or barriers to the student's occupational performance is important. The concern should be defined in these terms:

- *Alterable:* Performance can be changed.
- *Specific:* When and how long concern occurs.
- *Observable:* Performance can be seen.
- *Measurable:* Can be measured by various strategies such as counting or timing.

Instead of vague language (e.g., "Jill can't go to the bathroom by herself"), using specific language allows more information about the student's performance (e.g., "Jill can push her pants down before toileting, but an adult has to pull them up"). The concern (Jill can't pull up her pants) indicates a performance that can be changed, and the time it takes Jill to perform this activity can be observed and counted. Describe what would be an example of Jill doing this (e.g., pulling up her pants without twisting her pants, doing the task independently) and nonexamples (e.g., pulling up pants part of the way, twisting her pants so seams are not in correct area, not completing the task independently). Examples and nonexamples are specific to each student's needs.

STEP 2. SELECT THE MEASUREMENT STRATEGY

Next, what is problematic about the student's performance must be determined. Recording problematic performance depends on the concern (e.g., time or frequency of performance):

- *Duration (i.e., length of time):* Does the problematic performance happen too long (e.g., student is the last one to get dressed for recess) or too short (e.g., attention to task)?
- *Frequency (increase or decrease performance):* Does it happen too much (hits other students) or too little (eats only 2 bites at lunch)?
- *Accuracy (does not happen correctly):* Does the student require assistance (e.g., physical, verbal) to complete the task (e.g., minimal, moderate, or maximum assistance)?

Materials

Materials used for collecting baseline data could be a permanent product (e.g., classroom papers or journal, teacher's record book, student portfolio, Fitbit, word count tool, app-generated summaries) or an observation record (e.g., number of bites eaten, number of times a student is hit, number of seconds a student is out of his or her seat, task analysis checklist). The observation record could be a formal document or a piece of masking tape used to record the information and then attached to a sheet of paper.

Setting

The setting in which the data will be collected is generally the environment in which the concern occurs in the natural routine of the day. If the problematic performance occurs in more than one environment, data should initially be collected in several settings.

Reliability

Data must be reliable and valid. If more than one person collects the data, they should establish interrater reliability. The measurement strategy may consist of recording the amount of time it takes Jill to pull up her pants during toileting. If she is unable to complete the task because of physical or intellectual concerns, the amount of assistance needed may be measured.

STEP 3. DETERMINE CURRENT LEVEL OF PERFORMANCE (BASELINE)

Using the measurement strategy from Step 2, at least 3 stable data point are collected that are typical of the student's performance. If data are not stable (e.g., counts are 3, 10, 18), additional data may need to be collected. These data are summarized (the median is used because outlier data are disregarded) and compared with a performance standard.

Common performance standards in schools include peer performance, teacher expectations, school policy/standards, developmental norms, medical standards, expert judgment,

local norms, and criteria for this or the next environment. Sometimes local norms or expectations can be used (e.g., during the winter quarter, first graders will write at least 3 words and 20 letters, no hitting is allowed at school, all work must be completed within the class period). Sometimes the most appropriate standard is to compare the student's performance with that of classroom peers. Collect data from 3 "average" peers using the identified measurement strategy (*average* being defined as students performing in the middle range of this activity, not the highest or lowest performers). An example is included in Exhibit 2.1.

After the student's baseline performance data have been collected, they are compared with the standard. If there is no discrepancy, stop. If there is a discrepancy, consider whether it is large enough to warrant an intervention or whether another strategy is more appropriate. In the case presented in Exhibit 2.1, there is a significant discrepancy between the performance of Camden and his peers (0 words vs. a median of 5 words; 3 letters vs. a median of 19 letters).

STEP 4. SET THE GOAL

Consider the student's current performance (i.e., baseline) and standard (i.e., expected performance). For Camden, the team may write a student IEP goal to reflect what will be expected at the end of the year, for example, "By April 17, 2017, during 15 minutes of journal writing, Camden will write at least 5 words and 23 letters, independently, with letters formed according to curriculum and placed correctly on the line."

Exhibit 2.1. COMPARING STUDENT AND PEER PERFORMANCE

Area of concern: **Camden's** writing; independent writing in a journal was targeted by team.
Measurement strategy: Compare Camden's last 3 journal entries and those from 3 average-performing peers. (*Note:* The teacher allows 15 min for journal writing daily.)
Data collection: Note that although Camden wrote letters, no spaces were present, so they could not be considered words.

ENTRIES	CAMDEN	PEER A	PEER B	PEER C
Entry 1	3 letters, 0 words	12 letters, 3 words	20 letters, 4 words	12 letters, 4 words
Entry 2	0 letters, 0 words	15 letters, 5 words	22 letters, 5 words	19 letters, 3 words
Entry 3	5 letters, 0 words	18 letters, 5 words	22 letters, 5 words	19 letters, 3 words
Median: Letters	0, 3, 5 = 3	12, 15, 18 = 15	20, 22, 22 = 22	12, 19, 19 = 19
Median: Words	0, 0, 0 = 0	3, 5, 5 = 5	4, 5, 5 = 5	4, 3, 3 = 3

STEP 5. SET UP A CHART

Information can be recorded on a chart to create a picture of the student's rate of progress. Label the vertical and horizontal axes. In this case, the vertical axis denotes the number of letters and words, and the horizontal axis lists the dates. It is critical that the horizontal axis always measures the same period of time (e.g., Wednesday to Wednesday, Monday to Monday) and that the vertical axis also has an equal number of spaces (e.g., increments of 2, 5, or whatever is appropriate).

Enter the baseline data point and the goal data point (at the end of the predetermined period). Draw a line (known as the *goal line*) that connects the baseline point and the goal point. The goal line allows the team to determine the effectiveness of the intervention. A chart with these components can be found in Figure 2.1. Because both words and letters are being measured, they are listed on the same chart. Using two separate charts to document these data is also an option.

As seen in the figure, the baseline and 5 weeks of data collected during the intervention were recorded in dashes (number of words) and dots (number of letters). The baseline for Camden was 0 words, and his IEP goal is 5 words by April 17, so a black line was used to connect these points. This goal line illustrates the rate of progress that must be made for Camden to meet his goal. The same was done for letter data on the chart. Services begin with data gathered and entered either during each session or documented in a service log and added later. Figure 2.1 has baseline data as well as data for 5 weeks to demonstrate use of graphing.

STEP 6. DEVELOP A DECISION-MAKING PLAN FOR USE DURING SERVICE

Data should be collected regularly and at least once a week. Some data may be collected more frequently, for example, aggressive behavior or problems with swallowing foods would be monitored at a higher frequency than would putting on a coat or writing in a journal. A decision-making plan may be written as follows: "Data will be collected and graphed weekly by the teachers or occupational therapist during the natural routine of the day. Every 4 weeks, the occupational therapist and teachers will review the student's performance." The four-point decision-making rule may be used for decisions (see Figure 2.2):

- *Ascending goal lines:* If 4 consecutive data points fall above the goal line, the intervention is effective. If 4 consecutive data points fall below the goal line, the intervention is not effective; changes should be made to the intervention. If 4 consecutive data points fall above and below the goal line, continue with the current intervention.
- *Descending goal lines:* If 4 consecutive data points fall below the goal line, the intervention is effective. If 4 consecutive data points fall above the goal line, the intervention is not effective; changes should be made to the intervention. If 4 consecutive data points fall above and below the goal line, continue with the current intervention.

Figure 2.1.   SAMPLE OF PROGRESS MONITORING CHART WITH GOAL LINES

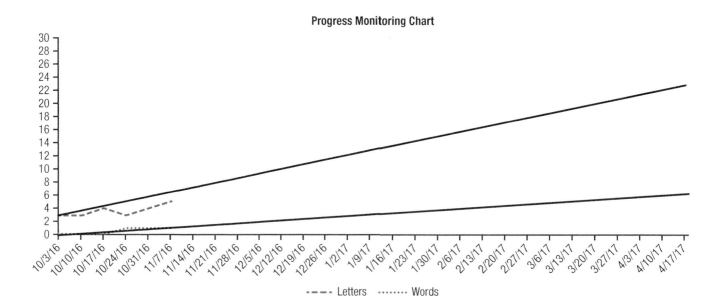

Figure 2.2. FOUR-POINT CONSECUTIVE DATA DECISION RULE

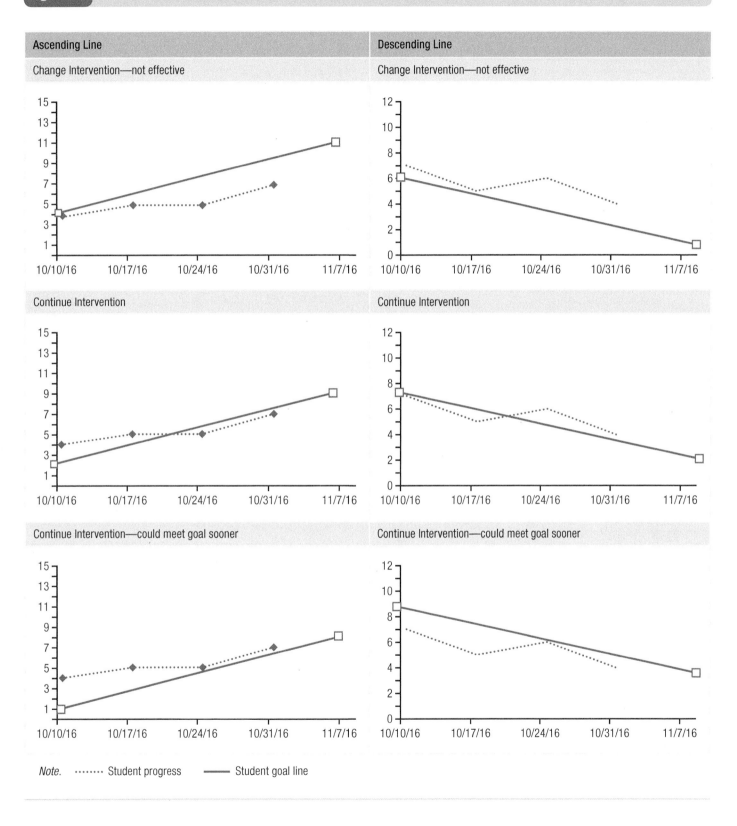

Note. ········ Student progress ——— Student goal line

FIDELITY OF IMPLEMENTATION (TREATMENT INTEGRITY)

When interpreting the effects of an intervention it is critical that the intervention was implemented as expected so the interpretation is accurate (Murphy & Gutman, 2012). If the protocol or sequence was not adhered to, the success of the intervention can be affected. Lack of fidelity of implementation makes it impossible to determine whether a lack of success is based on the student's performance or because the intervention was not implemented as established.

To ensure the intervention is implemented as intended (e.g., agreed on), written instructions, frequent monitoring to establish fidelity, and documentation of the intervention should be completed (Frolek Clark, 2013a). Exhibit 2.2 is a checklist that depicts the agreed-on activity and a place to chart each time the steps are carried out. Some weeks, because of school programs and fieldtrips, students may not be able to work on this activity. Having this noted on the form allows the team to determine whether the progress, or lack of progress, is due to opportunities to practice or something else.

Form 2.B, "Classroom Interventions: Effectiveness and Fidelity Rating Scale," is another example of a form that records fidelity of implementation. This classroom form is

---

Exhibit 2.2. CHECKLIST FOR MONITORING TREATMENT INTEGRITY IN PRESCHOOL

Student Name:____Mary Silver_____   School District: ____Maple Grove_____
Date:____November 7–11, 2016_____   Person Collecting Data:____Joanna Jones_____

Goal: Mary will be able to put on her coat, take off her own coat, and hang it on a hook, independently.
Teacher associate (TA):
1. Please put a ✓ in the box after completing the activity/exercise as demonstrated by the therapist.
2. Under Comments, note if Mary was I = *independent*, P = *physically assisted*, V = *verbally assisted*, or R = *refused assist*.
3. Each activity should be done daily as Mary arrives to or leaves school.

ACTIVITY	M	T	W	TH	F	COMMENTS
REMOVE AND HANG UP COAT						
1. TA will ask Mary to unzip her coat. If she does not respond within 10 seconds, provide verbal cue, "Pull the zipper down." If no response within 10 seconds, provide physical assistance to unzip coat.						
2. TA will ask Mary to remove her coat. If she does not respond within 10 seconds, provide verbal cue, "Pull out your arm." If no response within 10 seconds, provide physical assistance to remove coat.						
3. TA will ask Mary to hang up her coat. If she does not respond within 10 seconds, provide verbal cue, "Put your coat on the hook." If no response within 10 seconds, provide physical assistance to hang up coat.						
GET COAT OFF HOOK AND PUT COAT ON						
4. TA will ask Mary to get her coat. If she does not respond within 10 seconds, provide verbal cue, "Get your coat." If no response within 10 seconds, provide physical assistance to remove coat from hook.						
5. TA will ask Mary to put on her coat. If she does not respond within 10 seconds, provide verbal cue, "Pull your arm in." If no response within 10 seconds, provide physical assistance to put on coat.						
6. TA will ask Mary to zip her coat after the caregiver has put the tab in the zipper and pulled it up. If she does not respond within 10 seconds, provide verbal cue, "Pull the zipper up." If no response within 10 seconds, provide physical assistance to zip coat.						

Source. From "Using Data to Guide Your Decisions," by G. Frolek Clark, in H. Miller Kuhaneck and R. Watling (Eds.), *Autism: A Comprehensive Occupational Therapy Approach* (3rd ed.), Bethesda, MD: AOTA Press, p. 750. Copyright © 2010 by AOTA Press. Adapted with permission.

used by the teacher and occupational therapy practitioner to determine the consistency of implementation and to track the effectiveness of the intervention.

GOAL ATTAINMENT SCALING

Goal attainment scaling (GAS) is a method used in goal setting and monitoring. GAS can be used to identify client intervention outcomes that are relevant to families (Kiresuk, Smith, & Cardillo, 1994; Mailloux et al., 2007). Ottenbacher and Cusick (1990) described eight steps in the GAS process. Many of these are similar to the previously described steps for progress monitoring:

1. Identify the overall program goals for the client.
2. Identify problem areas.
3. Identify specific behaviors or events in problem areas that can be measured.
4. Determine how data will be collected.
5. Determine the expected level of performance.
6. Identify a continuum of outcomes (most to least favorable).
7. Review GAS to identify overlaps and gaps.
8. Determine when further evaluations will be conducted.

Schaaf and colleagues (2014) used GAS to demonstrate progress on a tooth brushing goal for a student and family (see Exhibit 2.3). The expected level of attainment is a score of 0, with scores of −1 and −2 indicating less and much less than expected level of attainment, respectively, whereas +1 and +2 indicate better and much better level of attainment than expected, respectively. The parent rates the child's goals after the intervention period (e.g., 10 weeks). For practitioners to effectively develop GAS, attending training courses is recommended.

RUBRICS

A *rubric* is a scoring tool that identifies the criteria for the student's performance and has gradations of quality for each of the criteria listed (Andrade, 1997). A rubric generally rates performance on a scale that ranges from excellent to poor. It clarifies the expectations and improves consistency and objectivity. Rubrics are created by

- Identifying the purpose,
- Describing baseline performance,
- Selecting performance components,
- Identifying a scale of measurement,
- Describing mastery criteria, and
- Describing criteria for each level of performance on the identified scale (Handley-More, 2008).

It is important to consider classroom standards and individualize mastery criteria for each student. Too often, expected points are arbitrarily assigned (e.g., 20 out of 25 points) without determining actual peer performance. Exhibit 2.4 provides an example of a rubric that was developed for a student in a third-grade classroom who was working on improving his handwriting legibility. The average student performance for his classroom was a total score of 17 out of 20.

RIOT/ICEL MATRIX

Considering several factors (e.g., ICEL: *i*nstruction, *c*urriculum, *e*nvironment, and *l*earner) when using methods to gather data (e.g., RIOT: *r*eview record, *i*nterview, *o*bserve, and *t*est) can facilitate participation and engagement in the

---

Exhibit 2.3. EXAMPLE OF GOAL ATTAINMENT SCALING

Goal: Decrease sensory sensitivity to the oral area as a basis for tooth brushing.
Current performance: It takes more than 20–30 minutes each day for tooth brushing with assistance from mother. Tooth brushing is unpleasant for **JH,** and often there is whining and crying.

−2 (much less than expected level of attainment)	Will brush teeth within a 17–20 minute time frame
−1 (less than expected level of attainment)	Will brush teeth within a 13–16 minute time frame
0 (expected level of attainment)	Will brush teeth within a 9–12 minute time frame
+1 (better than expected level of attainment)	Will brush teeth within a 5–8 minute time frame
+2 (much better than expected level of attainment)	Will brush teeth within a 1–4 minute time frame

Source. From "An Intervention for Sensory Difficulties in Children With Autism: A Randomized Trial," by R. Schaaf, T. Benevides, Z. Mailloux, P. Faller, J. Hunt, E. van Hooydonk, . . . D. Kelly, 2014, *Journal of Autism and Developmental Disorders*, Vol. 44, p. 1500. Copyright © 2014 by Springer. Reprinted with permission.

Exhibit 2.4. SAMPLE RUBRIC FOR HANDWRITING

Name: _____ My handwriting goal for today is _____ points.

☐ Check your spacing between words:
Rule: Leave enough room to write the letter "m" between any 2 words: big cat not: bigcat
Circle your score:

OOPS! I almost always forgot to follow the rule.	I remembered to follow the rule about half the time.	I remembered to follow the rule most of the time.	I always followed the rule.
1	2	3	4

☐ Check your spacing within words.
Rule: Leave no more than a skinny gap between the letters in a word: duck not: d u c k
Circle your score:

OOPS! I almost always forgot to follow the rule.	I remembered to follow the rule about half the time.	I remembered to follow the rule most of the time.	I always followed the rule.
1	2	3	4

☐ Check for floating letters.
Rule: All letters should touch the writing line: horse not: horse
Circle your score:

OOPS! I almost always forgot to follow the rule.	I remembered to follow the rule about half the time.	I remembered to follow the rule most of the time.	I always followed the rule.
1	2	3	4

☐ Check words with short letters: a, c, e, i, m, n, o, r, s, u, v, w, x, z
Rule: Short letters fill only about ½ of the width between the lines: fox not: FOX
Circle your score:

OOPS! I almost always forgot to follow the rule.	I remembered to follow the rule about half the time.	I remembered to follow the rule most of the time.	I always followed the rule.
1	2	3	4

☐ Check the words that have letters with tails: g, j, p, q, y
Rule: Letters with tails are short letters. They fill the bottom half of the line space and their tails go below the baseline: dog not: dog
Circle your score:

OOPS! I almost always forgot to follow the rule.	I remembered to follow the rule about half the time.	I remembered to follow the rule most of the time.	I always followed the rule.
1	2	3	4

Add up your score: _____ + _____ + _____ + _____ + _____ = _____

Did you meet your goal?   ☐ Yes   ☐ No

Source. Copyright © 2017 by Dottie Handley-More, Highline Public Schools, Washington. Used with permission.
Note. This rubric is intended to provide an example. Rubrics should be individualized based on the specific needs of the student and the teacher's expectations for classroom performance.

educational environment (Frolek Clark, Cahill, & Ivey, 2015). This framework organizes and documents data by including four information sources (review, interview, observe, test) with key domains of the educational environment (instruction, curriculum, environment, learner). The template (Form 2.C, "RIOT/ICEL Matrix") is included at the end of this chapter but was described more detail by Frolek Clark and colleagues (2015); this article is available in Appendix C, *School Practice Documentation: Documenting and Organizing Quantitative Data.*

FORMS: COLLECTING VALID AND RELIABLE DATA

Because data are used to make decisions about eligibility for programs, the need for related services, and progress toward the goals, it is critical that such data be gathered and recorded accurately to ensure reliable and valid measures. The next part of this section describes various forms to assist occupational therapy practitioners working in educational settings to collect various data.

GENERIC FORMS

Form 2.D, "Generic Data Collection Form," is a simple chart that can be used to collect data manually or electronically (using a spreadsheet with Microsoft Excel). The following are specific instructions on how to use this form:

- *"Date" column:* List all of the dates until the goal is reviewed (e.g., list each Monday or each Friday—there must be the same number of days between each of those cells).
- *"Baseline" column:* Enter the student's baseline (one number).
- *"Data Collected" column:* Enter data as they are collected during each therapy session or from another person who is recording the data.
- *"Goal" column (optional):* If you put the student's IEP goal data (e.g., 23 or 30) in this column, the points of the baseline data and these goal data will form the goal line (you have to connect it manually or electronically by inserting a line.

If you are using a spreadsheet, follow the steps to make a chart. This chart can be copied and pasted into reports.

Forms 2.E ("Ten-Trial Data Collection Form—Two Activities per Page") and 2.F ("Ten-Trial Data Collection Form—Long Form") are also generic charts that can be used to collect a variety of data, such as

- Number of times a student initiates social interaction within a (timed) 10-minute period. If the student initiates it more than 10 times, use the next row.
- Number of times a student correctly transitions 5 items from palm to fingertips. You can use a "+" for successful performance and a "0" or "−" if the student drops the items.
- Number of times a student successfully performs 10 trials during a prevocational experience (e.g., folded 10 towels, stapled first 10 packets). If you do not have 10 trials, just do not complete the last boxes.

You could use only Column 1 of these forms to record the time each week that a student needed to complete a task, attend during a 15-minute class period, or put on a coat. In that case, you would list the date and the number while leaving the other columns blank.

These forms can be used to create self-graphing documents through the following five steps:

1. Enter the data for each trial, using a "+" to indicate a trial when the student's performance meets the defined criteria and a "0" to indicate a trial when the student does not meet the defined criteria.
2. Count the number of "+" marks for the date, and enter the total in the column at the right.
3. Make an "X" on the line to the right of the trial number that corresponds to the total number of correct trials; for example, if the student's total is 6 correct trials, make an "X" on the line between Trial 6 and Trial 7.
4. Create the graph by drawing lines to connect the "X"s (see Exhibit 2.5).
5. If you are unable to collect data for all 10 trials, enter the total as a fraction (the number of correct trials over the total number of trials), and then calculate the percentage of correct trials (see the entry for 11/7/16 in Exhibit 2.5).

COLLECTING DATA ON SPECIFIC ACTIVITIES

Sometimes it is easier to use a form for specific activities (e.g., number of alphabet letters written) so you can quickly identify areas of strength and need. Form 2.G, "Data Collection Form— Alphabet," can be used to collect data on upper- or lowercase letters that the student is able to identify, imitate, copy, or write from dictation. You can dictate the letters out of order or use the data to record the student's work on classroom papers. At the bottom of the form, the data can be summarized. The last cell can be used to initialize who collected the data given that sometimes multiple people use this form in the classroom to collect data on one student.

When collecting data on numbers, Form 2.H, "Data Collection Form—Numbers," can be used. This form provides a quick reference on the numbers the student can identify, imitate, copy, or write from dictation.

COLLECTING DATA ON MULTIPLE GOALS

When a student has multiple goals, an efficient method of data collection is to place several goals on one data sheet, such as Form 2.I, "Documenting Multiple Goals." Form 2.J, "Documenting Multiple Goals on One Data Sheet: Sample," is a sample of Form 2.I, providing three different IEP goals for Kim, a student with significant needs. This form could remain in the classroom to allow various members of the IEP team to document the data collected on the goals (e.g., activating toys, all done, various work tasks).

Data can then be reviewed by the team to determine effectiveness of interventions. The number of columns for each goal is based on the number of trials used in the mastery criteria identified by the IEP team. The form also provides spaces to record the different activities so that the team can determine whether the student has generalized the skills to multiple activities. For this student, the team chose not to track

---

Exhibit 2.5. SELF-GRAPHING FORM EXAMPLE

Goal: CJ will independently fold and stack towels in 90% of trials.

DATE	1	2	3	4	5	6	7	8	9	10	TOTAL
10/3/16	0	0	+	0	0	+	0	+	+	0	4 (40%)
10/10/16	0	0	+	0	0	+	+	+	0	+	5 (50%)
10/17/16	0	+	+	+	0	0	+	+	+	+	7 (70%)
10/24/16	0	+	0	0	+	+	+	0	+	+	6 (60%)
10/31/16	+	+	0	+	+	0	+	+	+	0	7 (70%)
11/7/16	+	0	+	+	0	+	+	+			6/8 (75%)

Key:
+ = *towel folded independently.*
0 = *towel folded with verbal, gestural, or physical prompts.*

levels of prompts so performance was rated + *(independent)* or − *(needed prompting)*. However, the form could be easily modified to include the prompting hierarchy determined appropriate for the student and the task.

SUMMARY

Valid and reliable data are necessary for all decisions. Collecting quantitative data for decision making allows occupational therapists to document the effectiveness of their interventions and share these data with team members (including the family). Following the steps of data collection and measuring the fidelity of implementation are necessary for rigor in decision making.

REFERENCES

Andrade, H. G. (1997). Understanding rubrics. *Educational Leadership, 54*(4), 14–17.

Frolek Clark, G. (2010). Using data to guide your decisions. In H. M. Kuhaneck & R. Watling (Eds.), *Autism: A comprehensive occupational therapy approach* (3rd ed., pp. 743–776). Bethesda, MD: AOTA Press.

Frolek Clark, G. (2013a). Best practices in school occupational therapy documentation. In G. Frolek Clark & B. E. Chandler (Eds.), *Best practices for occupational therapy in schools* (pp. 107–119). Bethesda, MD: AOTA Press.

Frolek Clark, G. (2013b). Best practices in school occupational therapy intervention to support participation. In G. Frolek Clark & B. E. Chandler (Eds.), *Best practices for*

occupational therapy in schools (pp. 95–106). Bethesda, MD: AOTA Press.

Frolek Clark, G., Cahill, S., & Ivey, C. (2015). School practice documentation: Documenting and organizing quantitative data. *OT Practice, 20*(15), 12–15.

Frolek Clark, G., & Miller, L. (1996). Providing effective occupational therapy services: Data-based decision making in school-based practices. *American Journal of Occupational Therapy, 50,* 701–708. https://doi.org/10.5014/ajot.50.9.701

Handley-More, D. (2008). Developing and using rubrics in occupational therapy. *Journal of Occupational Therapy in Schools and Early Intervention, 1,* 24–32. https://doi.org/10.1080/19411240802060967

Handley-More, D., & Chandler, B. (2008). Occupational therapy decision-making process. In J. Jackson (Ed.), *Occupational therapy services for children and youth under IDEA* (3rd ed., pp 59–87). Bethesda, MD: AOTA Press.

Kiresuk, T. J., Smith, A. E., & Cardillo, J. E. (1994). *Goal attainment scaling: Applications, theory, and measurement.* Mahwah, NJ: Erlbaum.

Linder, J., & Clark, G. F. (2000). Best practices in documentation. In W. Dunn (Ed.), *Best practice occupational therapy* (pp. 135–145). Thorofare, NJ: Slack.

Mailloux, Z., May-Benson, T., Summers, C. A., Miller, L. J., Brett- Green, B., Burke, J. P., . . . Schoen, S. A. (2007). Goal attainment scaling as a measure of meaningful outcomes for children with sensory integration disorders. *American Journal of Occupational Therapy, 61,* 254–259. https://doi.org/10.5014/ajot.61.2.254

Murphy, S., & Gutman, S. (2012). Intervention fidelity: A necessary aspect of intervention effectiveness studies.

American Journal of Occupational Therapy, 66, 387–388. https://doi.org/10.5014/ajot.2010.005405

Ottenbacher, K. J., & Cusick, A. (1990). Goal attainment scaling as a method of clinical service evaluation. *American Journal of Occupational Therapy, 44,* 519–525. https://doi.org/10.5014/ajot.44.6.579

Schaaf, R., Benevides, T., Mailloux, Z., Faller, P., Hunt, J., van Hooydonk, E., . . . Kelly, D. (2014). An intervention for sensory difficulties in children with autism: A randomized trial. *Journal of Autism and Developmental Disorders, 44,* 1493–1506. https://doi.org/10.1007/s10803-013-1983-8

FORM 2.A. STEPS IN PROGRESS MONITORING

STEP	DESCRIPTION
1. Define the concern. Examples are "to drink," "to attend," "to handwrite." Operationalize by adding examples and nonexamples (i.e., what is acceptable and not acceptable).	"What" about behavior is problematic? Define behaviors so you can answer yes to the following questions: • *Alterable:* Can the behavior be changed? • *Specific:* Can you specify when or how the behavior occurs? • *Observable:* Can you see it occur? • *Measurable:* Can you specify a method of measuring it?
2. Select a measurement strategy.	Procedure you will use to collect the student's performance data. Should be systematic, reliable, valid, simple, efficient, and frequent. Dimensions of behavior: • *Frequency:* behavior happens too often or not often enough • *Duration:* behavior is too long or too short • *Latency:* after a prompt is given, behavior takes too long to begin. Determine: • How will data be collected? (e.g., observation, permanent product) • When and where will data be collected? (setting in which it occurs) • Who will collect the data? (i.e., reliability)
3. Document current level of performance (i.e., baseline).	For baseline, gather 3–4 data points over short time period. Data should be stable and represent typical behavior. Use median score. A standard is needed for comparison. Typical standards in education include teacher expectations; student expectations; criterion for the next environment; and school policy, standards, or benchmarks.
4. Set the goal. <table><tr><td>Conditions</td><td>Learner</td><td>Behavior</td><td>Criterion</td></tr><tr><td></td><td></td><td></td><td></td></tr></table>	Consider the defined behavior and the student's baseline and expected performance. • What are the conditions needed to achieve this behavior? • What is the criterion that shows mastery of this goal?
5. Set up a chart.	Create a graph. Excel works great, or use a paper graph. Add a goal line to connect baseline and expected behavior at the end of goal period.
6. Develop a decision-making plan.	This plan helps you remember to analyze the patterns of data on the chart. Data should be collected regularly. Examine data at least monthly. Decision rules (4-point) needs 4 consecutive data points to make a decision. • 4 consecutive data points above the goals line = *effective intervention.* • 4 consecutive data points below the goal line = *not working—change something.* • 4 consecutive data points above and below the goal line = *not consistent but seems to be responding—stay with current intervention.*

Source. Copyright © 2017 by Gloria Frolek Clark. Used with permission.

FORM 2.B. CLASSROOM INTERVENTIONS: EFFECTIVENESS AND FIDELITY RATING SCALE

The purpose of this form is to provide a way for an occupational therapy practitioner and teacher to track the effectiveness of classroom interventions and how consistently the interventions are implemented. Data from the form can be used to modify the interventions to better support behavior and ease of implementation.

DIRECTIONS:

1. Define the behavior of concern in the space below using specific, observable, and measureable terms.
2. Enter the behavior of concern in the space provided on the form.
3. Select an appropriate measurement strategy (e.g., duration, number of events, accuracy).
4. Create a rating scale based on the measurement strategy and enter values for each number on the scale.
5. Describe the classroom interventions (e.g., ball chair, visual schedule, movement break, assistive technology tool, handwriting checklist), including when and how to use them in the space provided at the bottom of the page.
6. Determine a schedule for completing the rating scale (e.g., at the end of each day, before each transition).

TO COMPLETE THE FORM: Circle or highlight the number that best matches your perception of the student's behavior during each rating period. Also circle or highlight your impression of how fully you have been able to implement each intervention (this is intended to help determine whether the interventions are a good match for the classroom environment).

Behavior: _____

Behaviors:	Rating Scale:	Date										
Behavior:	5 =		5	5	5	5	5	5	5	5	5	5
	4 =		4	4	4	4	4	4	4	4	4	4
	3 =		3	3	3	3	3	3	3	3	3	3
	2 =		2	2	2	2	2	2	2	2	2	2
	1 =		1	1	1	1	1	1	1	1	1	1
Interventions:	**Rating:**		**Rating/Total**									
Intervention 1	2 = *almost always* (>90%)		2	2	2	2	2	2	2	2	2	2
	1 = *frequently* (50%–90%)		1	1	1	1	1	1	1	1	1	1
	0 = *occasionally* (<50%)		0	0	0	0	0	0	0	0	0	0
Intervention 2	2 = *almost always* (>90%)		2	2	2	2	2	2	2	2	2	2
	1 = *frequently* (50%–90%)		1	1	1	1	1	1	1	1	1	1
	0 = *occasionally* (<50%)		0	0	0	0	0	0	0	0	0	0

Intervention 1: _____

Intervention 2: _____

FORM 2.C. RIOT/ICEL MATRIX

Directions: Place information gathered in the appropriate box. Not all of the boxes need to be filled, but gathered information should be sufficient for decision making.

MATRIX	INSTRUCTION (HOW IT IS BEING TAUGHT)	CURRICULUM (WHAT IS BEING TAUGHT)	ENVIRONMENT (WHERE IT IS BEING TAUGHT)	LEARNER (STUDENT)
Review (medical, educational, work experience)				
Interview (significant people, including family)				
Observe (in natural routines)				
Test or tools (linked to concerns and provide usable data)				

FORM 2.D. GENERIC DATA COLLECTION FORM

Directions: After entering the date and student's baseline and goal, record data in the third column. This could be done on a spreadsheet to generate an electronic chart.

DATE	BASELINE	DATA COLLECTED	GOAL

FORM 2.E. TEN-TRIAL DATA COLLECTION FORM—TWO ACTIVITIES PER PAGE

OCCUPATIONAL THERAPY DEPARTMENT
DATA COLLECTION FORM: 10 TRIALS (SHORT FORM)

STUDENT: _____ BIRTHDATE: _____

Directions: Enter the activity and, if it is timed, enter the amount of time allotted. Next, enter the date and complete the columns as needed. This form can be used to collect data for two activities.

ACTIVITY: _____ TIMED: _____

DATE	1	2	3	4	5	6	7	8	9	10	TOTAL

ACTIVITY: _____ TIMED: _____

DATE	1	2	3	4	5	6	7	8	9	10	TOTAL

FORM 2.F. TEN-TRIAL DATA COLLECTION FORM—LONG FORM

OCCUPATIONAL THERAPY DEPARTMENT
DATA COLLECTION FORM: 10 TRIALS (LONG FORM)

STUDENT: _____ BIRTHDATE: _____

Directions: Enter the activity and, if it is timed, enter the amount of time given. Next, enter the date and complete the columns as needed. This form collects data on 1–10 attempts on one line; two lines can be used for more than 10 attempts.

ACTIVITY: _____ TIMED: _____

DATE	1	2	3	4	5	6	7	8	9	10	TOTAL

FORM 2.G. DATA COLLECTION FORM—ALPHABET

OCCUPATIONAL THERAPY DEPARTMENT
Alphabet

STUDENT: _____ BIRTHDATE: _____

Directions: This form can be used for capital and lowercase letters (check the appropriate space below). Use "+" or "/" to indicate letters that the student writes correctly and "0" or "−" for errors. Note the method (i.e., imitated, copied, dictation). Person collecting data should initial in the space provided. If you use the form for both capital and lowercase letters, score them such as "+, −" for correct capital letter but incorrect lowercase letter.

Used for: Capital (uppercase) letters _____ Lowercase letters _____ Both _____

Date								
Method								
Initialed								
A a								
B b								
C c								
D d								
E e								
F f								
G g								
H h								
I i								
J j								
K k								
L l								
M m								
N n								
O o								
P p								
Q q								
R r								
S s								
T t								
U u								
V v								
W w								
X x								
Y y								
Z z								
TOTAL								

FORM 2.H. DATA COLLECTION FORM—NUMBERS

OCCUPATIONAL THERAPY DEPARTMENT
Numbers

STUDENT: _____ BIRTHDATE: _____

Directions: Use "+" or "/" to indicate numbers that the student writes correctly and "0" or "−" for errors. Note the method used (i.e., imitated, copied, dictation). The person collecting data should initial in the space provided.

Date								
Method								
Initial								
1								
2								
3								
4								
5								
6								
7								
8								
9								
10								
11								
12								
13								
14								
15								
16								
17								
18								
19								
20								
21								
22								
23								
24								
25								
TOTAL								

FORM 2.I. DOCUMENTING MULTIPLE GOALS

Directions: This form may be used to collect data on multiple goals. Complete the goal areas and student goals. Record data using the code below.

Student Name: _____   School Year: _____

Goal Area: _____

Goal:

Date:	1	2	3	4	5	6	7	8	9	10	Objects Used	Notes/Comments

+ = independent; − = requires prompting or physical assistance.

Goal Area: _____

Goal:

Date:	1	2	3	4	5	6	Center/Activity	Notes/Comments

+ = independent; − = requires prompting or physical assistance.

Goal Area: _____

Goal:

Date:	Task 1	Response	Task 2	Response	Task 3	Response	Notes/Comments

+ = independent; − = requires prompting or physical assistance.

FORM 2.J. DOCUMENTING MULTIPLE GOALS ON ONE DATA SHEET: SAMPLE

Student name: Kim T.   School Year: 2016–17

Activate Toys

Goal: When presented with a switch and a switch-activated toy or cause-and-effect game at the computer, Kim will push down on the switch to activate the toy or game from 2/10 trials to 9/10 trials.

Date:	1	2	3	4	5	6	7	8	9	10	Objects Used	Notes/Comments
10/4	−	−	+	−	+	−	−	−	+	−	Computer	Limited interest in fireworks game
10/11	−	−	−	+	+	−	+	+	+	−	Bubble Machine	Seemed to enjoy

+ = independent; − = requires prompting or physical assistance.

Using the "All Done" Box

Goal: During center activities, Kim will put away items used in an "all done" box when finished with each item from 1/6 items to 6/6 items.

Date:	1	2	3	4	5	6	Center/Activity	Notes/Comments
10/4	−	−	+	−	+	+	Writing center	
10/11	−	−	−	−	−	+	Writing center	Seemed agitated

+ = independent; − = requires prompting or physical assistance.

Completing Work Tasks

Goal: Given a 3-drawer work system, Kim will complete 3 work tasks independently with a prompt to initiate each work task during an independent work session from 1 work task per session to 3 work tasks per session.

Date:	Task 1	Response	Task 2	Response	Task 3	Response	Notes/Comments
10/6	Put-in (blocks)	+	3-shape puzzle	−	Jack-in-the-box	−	
10/13	Same	+	Same	−	Same	−	

+ = independent; − = requires prompting or physical assistance after being prompted to initiate the task.

Tiered Support:
Screening and Evaluation

Using a process of multiple steps to provide instruction and support for students struggling with academics and behavior has become common in educational systems. The number of tiers vary by state; however, a multitiered approach typically includes three levels of intensity of instruction or intervention. The first tier includes high-quality instruction available to all students. The second tier includes the first tier plus supplemental instruction or intervention. The third tier includes the previous tiers plus intensive instruction or intervention. The third and fourth tiers may include evaluation to determine the need for special education (SE).

Throughout this process, parental consent, team decisions, student performance data, and intervention or instruction are documented. As health care professionals with knowledge in areas such as physical (e.g., motor, sensory), cognitive, and social skills; mental health; literacy; technology; and environmental modifications, occupational therapists are often involved in this multitiered system of support. This chapter reviews a multitiered system of support (also known as *response to intervention [RtI]* or *early intervening services [EIS]*).

LANGUAGE DIFFERENCES IN MEDICAL AND EDUCATIONAL SETTINGS

Occupational therapy practitioners work in various settings, including medical and educational ones. State laws regulating licensure may contain language that seems different from language and practices in education. The language typically used in state regulatory laws requires an occupational therapist to conduct an evaluation before providing services and support; however, under the Individuals With Disabilities Education Improvement Act of 2004 (IDEA; P. L. 108–446), the term *evaluation* generally refers to an *evaluation for eligibility* (known as *full and individual initial evaluation* (§300.301[a]), and it is conducted if the child is suspected of having a disability, as defined by IDEA.

Occupational therapy practitioners are required to follow the language and process in their state practice act as well as in federal and state laws. To sort through some of the discrepancies between education and medical settings, it is important to understand the intent or purpose of the activity being requested. In an educational setting, a teacher may want some ideas to assist a student in (GE; i.e., screening) but may call it a "referral for occupational therapy." Likewise, a teacher may think that a student needs occupational therapy services but contacts the therapist to "see if Stella needs occupational therapy." The language can be confusing, but occupational therapists nevertheless must be clear on the intent of their actions and what is being requested. In many cases, an occupational therapy evaluation may be required even when a full evaluation under IDEA is not.

determine appropriate instructional strategies. Education laws consider identification for and provision of EIS (also known as *RtI* and *multitiered systems of support*) not an evaluation of eligibility for SE but a different process to determine the need for additional academic or behavioral supports to succeed in GE. States and local agencies are required to document the evaluation process, beginning with a signed parent request for a full and individual initial evaluation through the completion of the individualized education program (IEP) and parent-signed consent for services (see Table 3.1).

The purpose of IDEA is to "prepare a child for further education, employment and independent living" (§1400[d][I][A]), whereas the role of occupational therapy in schools is to "support the student's participation in his or her education program" (§1400[d][I][A][II][aa]). Table 3.2 identifies some of the reasons why an occupational therapist's services are requested. Note the critical differences between *Child Find*, a requirement of all school districts to identify and evaluate children to determine whether they may need special education (1412[a][3]), and *EIS*, a service school districts may provide to children who have not been identified as needing SE or related services but who may need additional academic and behavioral support (1413[f]).

EIS AND SCREENING IN GE

IDEA and the Every Student Succeeds Act of 2015 (P. L. 114–95) permit professionals, such as occupational therapists, to provide services to students in GE. For example, IDEA's EIS (§1413[f]) allows "evaluation, services, and supports" of students in GE to

INITIATING THE PROCESS

Requests for occupational therapy may come from parents, teachers, or other professionals. The occupational therapist has the responsibility of clarifying the purpose of the request. Examples of these requests can be found in Table 3.3.

Table 3.1.   FORMS REQUIRED UNDER IDEA FOR THE IEP EVALUATION PROCESS

FORM AND IDEA REFERENCE	PURPOSE
Request for full and individual initial evaluation (34 CFR §300.301)	Documents the request for initial evaluation to determine whether the child has a disability.
Excusal form (34 CFR §300.321[e])	Documents parental consent to excuse a member of the IEP team from attending an IEP meeting.
Determination of eligibility (34 CFR §300.311)	Documentation of eligibility is required (e.g., basis for determination); many states include this on the IEP forms.
IEP (34 CFR §300.321)	Documents the student's strengths and needs, current performance, and decisions made by the IEP team, including the student's proposed or current educational program, annual goals, services, modifications and supports, and participation with children without disabilities.

Note. IDEA = Individuals with Disabilities Education Improvement Act of 2004; IEP = individualized education program.

Table 3.2. PURPOSE OF OCCUPATIONAL THERAPY SERVICES UNDER TIERED SUPPORTS (SCREENING THROUGH INTERVENTION)

TIERED SUPPORTS	IDEA	OCCUPATIONAL THERAPY PROFESSION
Overview	*EIS:* Provide local education agencies up to 15% of SE monies per fiscal year (unless the district must maintain funds because of disproportionality and overidentification) to be used for children who are at risk academically and behaviorally. Activities may include • Professional development • Educational and behavioral evaluations, services, and support (§1413[f][2][B]).	"Occupational therapy addresses the physical, cognitive, psychosocial, sensory, and other aspects of performance in a variety of contexts to support engagement in everyday life activities that affect health, well-being, and quality of life" (AOTA, 2007, p. 3). Clients include persons, groups, and populations. Services may be provided directly to clients or indirectly on behalf of clients' (AOTA, 2014).
Tier 1: Screening for GE instruction and curriculum	*EIS—rule of construction:* Screening of a student by a teacher or specialist to determine appropriate instructional strategies for curriculum implementation shall not be considered an evaluation for eligibility for SE and related services (§1414[a][1][E], §300.302).	Obtaining and reviewing data relevant to a potential client to determine the need for further evaluation and intervention (AOTA, 2015). If allowable under state regulatory law and agency policy, may provide screening to determine appropriate GE strategies. May provide general information and professional development to educators to enhance performance in GE. *Note.* At any time, if a student is suspected of having a disability, the occupational therapist must consider evaluation (which aligns with state and federal Child Find requirements).
Tier 2: Supplemental or Tier 3: Intensive interventions	*Supplemental or intensive interventions in GE:* If a child suspected of having a learning disability participated in a scientific, research-based intervention, then the strategies used and data collected must be documented, and parents must be provided documentation about the state's policies regarding this process (§300.311). (*Note.* Supplemental interventions may be additional activities for practice or learning; intensive interventions may include one-to-one work using various strategies and may require an occupational therapy evaluation.)	The OT may assist teachers in identifying general activities to assist the population. If allowable under state regulatory law and agency policy, the OT may provide episodic assistance or short-term interventions to enhance GE performance. *Note.* At any time, if a student is suspected of having a disability, the OT must consider evaluation (which aligns with state and federal Child Find requirements).
Tier 4: Evaluation for SE and related services	*Is this a child with a disability?* *Child Find:* All children living in the state who have disabilities (e.g., homeless, wards of the state, attending private schools) and who are in need of SE and related services must be identified, located, and evaluated. Children who are suspected of having a disability and in need of SE must be identified (§300.111[c][1]). *Full and individual initial evaluation:* The team must determine whether child has a disability, his or her educational needs as well as present levels of academic achievement and related developmental needs, whether SE and related services are needed, and whether any additions or modifications are needed to meet the student's measurable annual goals (§300.305).	The process of obtaining and interpreting data necessary for intervention. This includes planning for and documenting the evaluation process and results (AOTA, 2015). Occupational therapy evaluation is part of determining eligibility and need for SE and related services (e.g., occupational therapy). "An occupational therapy evaluation should consider the student's occupational performance across the full range of settings he or she encounters during the school day, including classroom, hallways, lunchroom, playground, and other settings and should include all areas of occupation" (Coster & Frolek Clark, 2013, p. 85).

(Continued)

Table 3.2.   PURPOSE OF OCCUPATIONAL THERAPY SERVICES UNDER TIERED SUPPORTS (SCREENING THROUGH INTERVENTION) *(CONT.)*

TIERED SUPPORTS	IDEA	OCCUPATIONAL THERAPY PROFESSION
Tier 4: SE student intervention services	*Does this child with a disability need SE and related services?* *SE:* Designed to meet the child's unique needs and prepare the child for further education, employment, and independent living (§1400). *Related services:* Designed to enable a child with a disability to receive a free appropriate public education, as described in the IEP; may be required to assist a child with a disability to benefit from SE (§1401[26]). *Types of services:* The IEP will contain a statement of SE and related services and supplementary aids and services, provided to the child, or on behalf of the child, and a statement of program modifications or supports for school personnel (§1414[d]).	Use professional and clinical reasoning, evidence-based practice, and therapeutic use of self to implement the most appropriate types of interventions (AOTA, 2015). Types of intervention may include occupations and activities, preparatory methods and tasks, education and training, advocacy, and group interventions (AOTA, 2014). Occupational therapy practitioners may provide the following services in schools: • Hands-on services with team supports (provided to the child) • Team supports (on behalf of the child) • System supports (Hanft & Shepherd, 2016).

Note. AOTA = American Occupational Therapy Association; EIS = early intervening services; FAPE = free appropriate public education; GE = general education; IDEA = Individuals with Disabilities Education Improvement Act of 2004; IEP = individualized education program; OT = occupational therapist; SE = special education.

Table 3.3.   EXAMPLES OF REQUESTS FOR OCCUPATIONAL THERAPY SERVICES

REQUEST	ACTION: IF OT IS NOT ALLOWED TO COLLECT INFORMATION ON A SPECIFIC STUDENT BEFORE EVALUATION FOR SE	ACTION: IF OT IS ALLOWED TO COLLECT INFORMATION ON A SPECIFIC STUDENT BEFORE EVALUATION FOR SE
GE: Screening to assist in identifying appropriate GE strategies to enhance performance.	Any screening activities should be documented, even if the OT is providing general information to the classroom teacher (not specific to a student).	Any screening activities should be documented.
Child Find: Assistance to determine whether a child in GE should be referred for an occupational therapy evaluation as part of the full and individual initial evaluation under IDEA.	Provide the teacher with information (e.g., equipment, child development); provide information about appropriate referrals for occupational therapy services under IDEA.	If the parents have been notified by the school and agree to occupational therapy assistance, the OT may observe the student in the school environment.
SE: Assistance to determine whether the child with a disability who is receiving SE services could benefit from occupational therapy.	Provide the teacher with information (e.g., equipment, child development); provide information about appropriate referrals for occupational therapy services under IDEA.	If the parents have been notified by the school and agree to occupational therapy observation, observe the student in the school environment. Parental consent for occupational therapy evaluation should be sought if there are data to indicate evaluation is necessary.
SE (supports to the teacher): Assistance with training, modifications, or equipment needs (e.g., the child may have received occupational therapy services in the past but they were discontinued; teacher is requesting assistance).	Provide the teacher with information (e.g., equipment, child development); provide information about appropriate referrals for occupational therapy services under IDEA.	If the parents have been notified by the school and agree to occupational therapy team support, the OT may observe the student in the school environment. Parental consent for occupational therapy evaluation should be sought if there are data to indicate evaluation is necessary.

Note. Parental agreement must be obtained in accordance with district and agency procedures. GE = general education; IDEA = Individuals with Disabilities Education Improvement Act of 2004; OT = occupational therapist; SE = special education.

Occupational therapy practitioners should remember to refer to their state regulatory laws and agencies' policies regarding practices in their state. Once a student is suspected of having a disability, parental consent for an occupational therapy evaluation under IDEA (either as part of a full and individual initial evaluation or after the student has been found to be eligible for SE) should be sought.

The *Guidelines for Documentation of Occupational Therapy* (American Occupational Therapy Association [AOTA], 2013) indicates that the referral source and the reason for referral to occupational therapy screening or evaluation should be documented. These data may be collected by each individual occupational therapist or by someone overseeing referrals to the occupational therapy department. Form 3.A, "Documentation of Referral Sources," provides this information as well as the student's demographic information and the outcome of the referral. Using numbers (e.g., codes such as 1 = *parent/family*, 2 = *principal*, 3 = *GE teacher*) allows the data to be easily entered on a worksheet and tabulated. To maintain the confidentiality of students being referred, we do not recommend that this completed form be available across all occupational therapists in the department but instead be limited to the appropriate personnel.

SUPPORT FOR GE TEACHERS

Sometimes the teacher requests support to facilitate learning or performance in the classroom. Forms 3.B, "Sample Form for Request for Occupational Therapy Support—Teacher," and 3.C, "Sample Form for Request for Occupational Therapy Support—Consultation for Student," provide a record of teacher concerns and allow the occupational therapist to document the contact. Form 3.B documents supports to the teacher and should be used in states where licensure or educational policy does not allow contact with students before obtaining the parent's consent for evaluation (see Table 3.3).

Form 3.C can be used in states where occupational therapists can work with GE teachers and at-risk students in the GE program. This form documents information from the teacher about the student. District and agency policies regarding parent notification and consent must be followed. Working with the teacher and student allows the occupational therapist to collect data and assist in GE interventions. If a student does not respond to these supports and interventions, Child Find would require that he or she be considered for a full and individualized evaluation, per parent consent.

EVALUATION TO DETERMINE NEED FOR SE

When the process has moved to an evaluation for IDEA services, completion of the occupational profile (AOTA, 2014) initiates the data collection process by gaining a better understanding about the student. This process may be accomplished through record review, interviews, and observation. Sometimes it is helpful to have a document that can provide occupational therapists with questions to ask and a place to document the answer. The purpose of the interview form (see Form 3.D, "Questions for Interviewing Parent and Teacher") is to gain a better understanding of the student and his or her performance during the educational program. Parents, teachers, and the student may have data necessary for decision making and should be interviewed to gather information to use when making decisions about eligibility and program needs.

INTERVIEWING

Interviewing a student often provides insight into the supports and barriers in the educational day. A sample form for a student interview is provided in Form 3.E, "Questions for Interviewing Students."

REVIEWING RECORDS, INTERVIEWING, OBSERVATION, AND RECORDING TEST DATA

Form 3.F, "Documentation Template Using RIOT," can be used by occupational therapists documenting data collection. Screening all occupations is important so that areas that require more in-depth evaluation can be identified. Sections for documenting information collected from record review, interviews, observation, and tests and tools are provided. Although many additional areas are included, only the areas that are problematic would require observation or further interview. The "Notes" area on the last page of Form 3.F can be used to document contact with the teachers, parents, students, and others. When a new request for occupational therapy is received, this form can be used as the first step to record all of the data.

OBSERVATION

Observation of the student in the environment where the concern occurs and while it is occurring is necessary to understand the student–occupation–environment fit. This approach provides opportunities to observe the supports and barriers in the environment as well as the student's instruction and curriculum. These data can be used as the baseline when establishing goals and reporting progress. In addition, gathering quantitative data of peers' performance provides insight into educational requirements (or for young students, developmental expectations) and can be used to determine the student's discrepancy from peers.

In addition to the multiple data collection forms for quantitative data found in Chapter 2, this text includes a form that can be used for comments about the context and environment, teacher supports, task supports and activity demands, and performance skills and patterns on the basis of the *Occupational Therapy Practice Framework: Domain and Process* (AOTA, 2014) as well as evidence-based Tier 1 classroom behavioral supports (Simonsen, Fairbanks, Briesch, Myers, & Sugai, 2008; see Form 3.G, "Occupational Performance Observations"). Form 3.H, "Sensory Processing Observations," provides a record of observations by the occupational therapist during the student's participation in the natural school environment. Form 3.I, "Example of a Completed Sensory Processing Observations Form," provides an example of how the form was completed to support tiered behavioral interventions for a GE kindergarten student in a dual-language program.

SOCIAL PARTICIPATION

One of the occupations within the domain of occupational therapy is social participation. When a student's social interactions are inappropriate, assistance from an occupational therapy practitioner is sometimes requested. Occupational therapy practitioners collaborate with other professionals (e.g., psychologists, social workers, school counselors, staff certified in applied behavior analysis) to address social skills and behavior problems (Hanft & Shepherd, 2016). Some schools have criteria on when to conduct a *functional behavioral assessment*, which is a procedure to define a student's behavior and determine its cause. Some teams may start with the *ABC Model of Behavior,* which is used to record what happened (*antecedent*), what the student did (*behavior*), and what happened next (*consequence*).

Form 3.J, "Gathering ABC Data," can be used during an interview or observation to assist with decision making. We added a column for environment because the environment may influence performance (e.g., accidental pushing in busy hallway, loud noises in gym). An example of how to use this form is provided in Form 3.K, "Sample of ABC Data."

ASSESSMENT TOOLS

Assessment tools should be used with the population and intent for which they were developed. In addition, occupational therapists may use tools that were normed in the school district or state. The evaluation tools listed in Table 3.4 have been sorted by the domain of occupational therapy.

ANALYZING DATA AND MAKING DECISIONS

Occupational therapists conduct the evaluation, analyze the data, and then complete a report that describes the student's current performance; identifies the impact of the student's disability on his or her involvement and progress in the educational program (or participation in appropriate activities for preschoolers); and describes what the student needs to learn (curriculum), the best methods for learning this information (instruction), and any environmental modifications for learning. "Occupational therapy practitioners working in public education settings focus on supporting students in their educational program, which include[s] an understanding of the school district's academic and functional curriculum and preparing students for postsecondary life" (Frolek Clark, 2016, p. 180).

Students who are eligible for SE services do not have to qualify for additional services. After the needs, educational placement, and student goals have been determined, the team decides what services are necessary to meet those student goals. Data gathered during the evaluation process should assist the occupational therapist in determining whether occupational therapy should be suggested for a student. To answer the question, "Does this student need occupational therapy services to benefit from his or her educational program?" the occupational therapist should consider the following factors:

- Does this problem currently affect the student's ability to benefit from or participate in his or her educational program (including academic and nonacademic activities)?
- Have other documented attempts been made to improve performance?
- Is the potential for change in the student's goal or performance through intervention feasible (e.g., changes are unrelated to maturity)?
- Are the concerns within the domain of occupational therapy?
- To meet the student's needs, is specialized instruction from an occupational therapist required? (Note that assistance in modifying the environment or training others could be accomplished through services on behalf of the child or support to educational staff.)

A recommendation of therapy may be made; however, decisions are made at the IEP meeting after determination of eligibility and the educational program. Form 3.L, "Sample of an Occupational Therapy Report Template," offers a sample template for a report.

Examples of completed evaluation forms are provided to assist occupational therapists in understanding the many possible ways to state information. Form 3.M, "Sample Evaluation Report," is the template from Form 3.L, completed

Table 3.4. SAMPLE ASSESSMENTS USED BY OCCUPATIONAL THERAPISTS IN SCHOOLS

DOMAIN OF OCCUPATIONAL THERAPY	ASSESSMENT
Areas of occupation	Adaptive Behavior Assessment System–School (3rd ed.; Harrison & Oakland, 2015)
	Canadian Occupational Performance Measure (4th ed.; Law et al., 2005)
	Children's Assessment of Participation and Enjoyment and Preferences for Activities of Children (King et al., 2005)
	Children's Occupational Self-Assessment (Keller et al., 2005)
	DeCoste Writing Protocol (DeCoste, 2014)
	Evaluation Tool of Children's Handwriting (Amundson, 1995)
	Functional Evaluation for Assistive Technology (Raskind & Bryant, 2002)
	Miller Function and Participation Scales (Miller, 2006)
	Minnesota Handwriting Assessment (Reisman, 1999)
	Pediatric Evaluation of Disability Inventory–Computer Adaptive Test (2nd ed.; Haley et al., 2012)
	Perceived Efficacy and Goal Setting System (Missiuna, Pollock, & Law, 2004)
	Preschool Play Materials Preference Inventory (Wolfberg, 1995)
	Protocol for Accommodation in Reading (DeCoste & Wilson, 2012)
	Revised Knox Preschool Play Scale (Knox, 2008)
	Roll Evaluation of Activities of Daily Living (Roll & Roll, 2014)
	School AMPS (Fisher et al., 2005)
	School Function Assessment (Coster et al., 1998)
	School Setting Interview (Hemmingsson et al., 2005)
	Test of Handwriting Skills–Revised (Milone, 2007)
	The Print Tool (Olsen & Knapton, 2016)
	Vineland Adaptive Behavior Scales (2nd ed.; Sparrow et al., 2005)
	Vocational Fit Assessment (Persch et al., 2015)
Performance skills	Battelle Developmental Inventory (2nd ed.; Newborg, 2004)
	Bruinicks–Oseretsky Test of Motor Proficiency (2nd ed.; Bruinicks & Bruinicks, 2005)
	Developmental Test of Visual Perception (3rd ed.; Hammill et al., 2013)
	Developmental Test of Visual Perception–Adolescent and Adult (Reynolds et al., 2002)
	Developmental Test of Visual–Motor Integration (6th ed.; Beery et al., 2010)
	Goal-Oriented Assessment of Lifeskills (Miller et al., 2013)
	Motor-Free Visual Perception Test (4th ed.; Colarusso & Hammill, 2015)
	Movement ABC–2 (Henderson et al., 2007)
	Peabody Developmental Motor Scales (2nd ed.; Folio & Fewell, 2000)
	Sensory Processing Measure (Miller-Kuhaneck et al., 2010)
	Sensory Profile–2; Sensory Profile–2 School Companion (2nd ed.; Dunn, 2014)
	Sensory Profile–Adolescent/Adult (Brown & Dunn, 2002)
Performance patterns	Canadian Occupational Performance Measure (4th ed.; Law et al., 2005)
	Children's Assessment of Participation and Enjoyment and Preferences for Activities of Children (King et al., 2005)
	Perceived Efficacy and Goal Setting System (Missiuna et al., 2004)
Context and environment	Canadian Occupational Performance Measure (4th ed.; Law et al., 2005)
	Children's Assessment of Participation and Enjoyment and Preferences for Activities of Children (King et al., 2005)
	Perceived Efficacy and Goal Setting System (Missiuna et al., 2004)

Note. Adapted from Tomchek & Koenig (2016) and Coster & Frolek Clark (2013). Used with permission.

with the data on a student who has difficulty participating in his educational program.

REEVALUATION TO DETERMINE CONTINUED ELIGIBILITY

Under IDEA, reevaluations must be conducted at least every 3 years to determine whether the child continues to have a disability (as defined by IDEA), to identify the child's educational and developmental needs, and to determine whether the child continues to be in need of SE and related services (34 CFR §300.305). The reevaluation also helps identify the present levels of academic achievement and whether there is a need for additional services or program modifications (34 CFR §300.305).

The occupational therapist's role in the reevaluation is similar to that in the initial evaluation. That role begins with updating the occupational profile and includes a record review, observations of occupational performance in relevant school contexts, interviews, and, if needed, standardized assessment. Form 3.N, "Sample Reevaluation Report," provides an example of a comprehensive reevaluation report for Lettie, a student with autism spectrum disorder. Lettie recently moved to the district and was placed in a self-contained SE classroom on the basis of records received from the previous district. Standardized assessments were selected to address concerns identified by the IEP team and questions that remained unanswered after the occupational profile interviews and observations.

SUMMARY

Occupational therapists working in schools often collaborate with other professionals to identify GE students who are at risk, students who are suspected of having a disability (Child Find), and students who are eligible for Section 504 of the Rehabilitation Act of 1973 (P. L. 93–112; 2008; i.e., have a disability but do not need specialized instruction) or IDEA (i.e., meet one of the categories of educational disability and need specialized instruction). Data for making decisions should be gathered through multiple methods across the environments in which the concern occurs.

If the state educational agency and regulatory laws allow a multitiered system of support, occupational therapists work with GE teachers and students to enhance the ability of the student to participate in the GE program. Otherwise, occupational therapists can provide evidence-based support for teachers through professional development (e.g., presentation on fine motor development or self-regulation).

For students receiving a full and individual initial evaluation, or those who are in a SE program and have been referred for an occupational therapy evaluation, the occupational therapist synthesizes information gathered through the evaluation to make suggestions about the student's needs related to curricula (what the student needs to learn), instruction (how the student needs to learn this information), and environment (where the student needs to learn). The occupational therapist is an essential member of the student's IEP team and presents data to assist the team in making decisions about the student's strengths, needs, current level of functioning, and IEP goals and about services that will help the student meet those goals.

REFERENCES

American Occupational Therapy Association. (2007). *Model occupational therapy practice act.* Retrieved from http://www.aota.org/~/media/Corporate/Files/Advocacy/State/Resources/PracticeAct/MODEL%20PRACTICE%20ACT%20FINAL%202007.pdf

American Occupational Therapy Association. (2013). Guidelines for documentation of occupational therapy. *American Journal of Occupational Therapy, 67*(Suppl.), S32–S38. https://doi.org/10.5014/ajot.2013.67S32

American Occupational Therapy Association. (2014). Occupational therapy practice framework: Domain and process (3rd ed.). *American Journal of Occupational Therapy, 68*(Suppl. 1), S1–S48. https://doi.org/10.5014/ajot.2014.682006

American Occupational Therapy Association. (2015). Standards of practice for occupational therapy. *American Journal of Occupational Therapy, 69*(Suppl. 3), 1–6. https://doi.org/10.5014/ajot.2015.696S06

Amundson, S. (1995). *Evaluation Tool of Children's Handwriting.* Homer, AK: OT Kids.

Beery K., Buktenica, N. A., & Beery, N. (2010). *The Beery–Buktenica Developmental Test of Visual Motor Integration* (6th ed.). San Antonio: Pearson Assessments.

Brown, C., & Dunn, W. (2002). *Adolescent/Adult Sensory Profile.* San Antonio: Pearson Assessments.

Bruinicks, R. H., & Bruinicks, B. D. (2005). *Bruinicks–Oseretsky Test of Motor Proficiency* (2nd ed.). Circle Pines, MN: AGS.

Colarusso, R., & Hammill, D. (2015). *Motor-Free Visual Perception Test–4 (MVPT–4).* Novato, CA: Academic Therapy Publications.

Coster, W., Deeney, T., Haltwanger, J., & Haley, S. (1998). *The School Function Assessment.* San Antonio: Psychological Corporation.

Coster, W., & Frolek Clark, G. (2013). Best practices in school occupational therapy evaluation to support participation. In G. Frolek Clark & B. E. Chandler (Eds.), *Best practices for occupational therapy in schools* (pp. 83–93). Bethesda, MD: AOTA Press.

DeCoste, D. (2014). *The DeCoste Writing Protocol: Evidence-based research to make instructional and accommodation decisions.* Volo, IL: Don Johnston.

DeCoste, D., & Wilson, L. B. (2012). *Protocol for accommodations in reading* [e-book]. Volo, IL: Don Johnston.

Dunn, W. (2014). *Sensory Profile–2.* Bloomington, MN: Psychological Corporation.

Every Student Succeeds Act of 2015, Pub. L. 114–95, § 114 Stat. 1177

Fisher, A., Bryze, K., Hume, V., & Grinswold, L. (2005). *School AMPS: School version of the Assessment of Motor and Process Skills* (2nd ed.). Fort Collins, CO: Three Star Press.

Folio, R., & Fewell, R. (2000). *Peabody Developmental Motor Scales* (2nd ed.). Austin, TX: Pro-Ed.

Frolek Clark, G. (2016). Collaborating within the paces: Structures and routines. In B. Hanft & J. Shepherd (Eds.), *Collaborating for student success* (2nd ed., pp 177–207). Bethesda, MD: AOTA Press.

Haley, S. M., Coster, W. J., Dumas, H. M., Fragala-Pinkam, M. A., & Moed, R. (2012). *Pediatric Evaluation of Disabilities Inventory Computer Adaptive Test*. Retrieved from http://www.pedicat.com

Hammill, D., Pearson, N., & Voress, J. (2013). *Development Test of Visual Perception* (3rd ed.). Austin, TX: Pro-Ed.

Hanft, B., & Shepherd, B. (Eds.). (2016). *Collaborating for student success* (2nd ed.). Bethesda, MD: AOTA Press.

Harrison, P., & Oakland, T. (2015). *Adaptive Behavior Assessment System, Third Edition (ABAS–3)*. Torrance, CA: Western Psychological Services.

Hemmingsson, H., Egilson, S., Hoffman, O., & Kielhofner, G. (2005). *A user's manual for the School Setting Interview (SSI) Version 3*. Chicago: University of Illinois Press.

Henderson, S., Sugden, D., & Barnett, A. (2007). *Movement Assessment Battery for Children–Second Edition (Movement ABC–2)*. London: Harcourt Assessment.

Individuals with Disabilities Education Improvement Act of 2004, Pub L. 108–446, 20 U.S.C. §1400–1482.

Keller, J., Kafkes, A., Basu, S., Feerico, J., & Kielhofner, G. (2005). *Child Occupational Self-Assessment*. Chicago: University of Illinois at Chicago.

King, G., Law, M., King S., Hurley, P., Rosebaum, P., & Hanna, S. (2005). *Children's Assessment of Participation and Enjoyment (CAPE) and Preferences for Activities of Children (PAC)*. San Antonio: Harcourt.

Knox, S. (2008). Development and current use of the Revised Knox Preschool Play Scale. In L. Parham & L. Fazio (Eds.), *Play in occupational therapy for children* (pp. 55–70). St. Louis: Elsevier Health Sciences. https://doi.org/10.1016/B978-032302945-4.10003-0

Law, M., Baptiste, S., Carswell, A., McColl, M. A., Polatajko, H., & Pollock, N. (2005). *The Canadian Occupational Performance Measure* (4th ed.). Ottawa, Ontario: CAOT Publications.

Miller, L. J. (2006). *Miller Function and Participation Scales manual*. San Antonio: Pearson Assessments.

Miller, L. J., Oakland, T., & Herzberg, D. (2013). *Goal-Oriented Assessment of Lifeskills (GOAL)*. Torrance, CA: Western Psychological Services.

Miller-Kuhaneck, H., Henry, D., & Glennon, T. (2010). *Sensory Processing Measure—Main classroom and school environment forms*. Los Angeles: Western Psychological Services.

Milone, M. (2007). *Test of Handwriting Skills–Revised*. Novato, CA: Academic Therapy Publications.

Missiuna, C., Pollock, N., & Law, M. (2004). *Perceived Efficacy and Goal Setting System (PEGS)*. Oxford, England: Harcourt Assessment.

Olsen, J. Z., & Knapton, E. F. (2016). *The Print Tool* (5th ed.). Cabin John, MD: Handwriting Without Tears.

Newborg, J. (2004). *Battelle Developmental Inventory–Second Edition manual*. Rolling Meadows, IL: Riverside.

Persch, A. C., Gugiu, P. C., Onate, J. A., & Cleary, D. S. (2015). Development and psychometric evaluation of the Vocational Fit Assessment (VFA). *American Journal of Occupational Therapy, 69*, 1–8. https://doi.org/10.5014/ajot.2015.019455

Raskind, M., & Bryant, B. (2002). *Functional Evaluation for Assistive Technology (FEAT): Examiners manual*. Austin, TX: Psycho-Educational Services.

Reisman, J. E. (1999). *The Minnesota Handwriting Assessment user's manual*. San Antonio: Psychological Corporation.

Reynolds, C. R., Pearson, N. A., & Voress, J. K. (2002). *Developmental Test of Visual Perception–Adolescent and Adult (DTVP–A)*. Lutz, FL: Psychological Assessment Resources.

Roll, K., & Roll, W. (2014). *Roll Evaluation of Activities of Daily Life*. San Antonio: Pearson.

Section 504 of the Rehabilitation Act of 1973, Pub. L. 93–112, as amended 29 U.S.C. § 1794 (2008).

Simonsen, B., Fairbanks, S., Briesch, A., Myers, D., & Sugai, G. (2008). Evidence-based practices in classroom management: Considerations for research to practice. *Education and Treatment of Children, 31*(3), 351–380.

Sparrow, S. S., Cicchetti, D. V., & Balla, D. A. (2005). *Vineland Adaptive Behavior Scales* (2nd ed.). San Antonio: Pearson Assessments.

Tomchek, S., & Koenig, K. P. (2016). *Occupational therapy practice guidelines: Individuals with autism spectrum disorder*. Bethesda, MD: AOTA Press.

Wolfberg, P. J. (1995). Enhancing children's play. In K. A. Quill (Ed.), *Teaching children with autism: Strategies to enhance communication and socialization* (pp. 193–217). Independence, KY: Thomson Delmar Learning.

FORM 3.A. DOCUMENTATION OF REFERRAL SOURCES

DOCUMENTATION OF NEW SCREENINGS AND EVALUATIONS

School Year: _____

Therapist: _____   School District: _____

Directions: Enter data as new referrals are made. Codes are listed below:

Column	Description or Codes
1–Last name	Enter student's last name.
2–First name	Enter student's first name.
3–School code	Enter school code. 1 = Jefferson Elementary; 2 = Roosevelt Elementary; 3 = Lincoln Middle School; 4 = Kennedy High School.
4–Grade	Enter code. PS = preschool; K = kindergarten; G1 = Grade 1; G2 = Grade 2, and so on.
5–Referred by	Enter code. 1 = parent or family; 2 = principal; 3 = GE teacher; 4 = SE teacher; 5 = psychologist; 6 = consultant; 7 = other.
6–Reason	Enter code. 1 = evaluation for SE; 2 = screening; 3 = request for support to teacher.
7–Concern (may list more than one)	Enter code. *Self-care:* 1 = dressing; 2 = feeding or eating; 3 = hygiene, grooming, or toileting. *Education:* 4 = access and participation; 5 = attention; 6 = literacy–writing; 7 = literacy–reading; 8 = functional motor skills (e.g., cutting, coloring); 9 = organization; 10 = prevocation. *Other:* 11 = play or leisure; 12 = social participation; 13 = other: describe in 1–3 words.
8–Outcome	Enter code. 1 = evaluation conducted, student not eligible for SE; 2 = evaluation conducted, student eligible, OT on IEP; 3 = evaluation conducted, student eligible, no OT on IEP; 4 = evaluation conducted, 504 written; 5 = no evaluation conducted.

#	Last name	First name	School	Current grade	Referred by	Reason	Concern	Outcome
1								
2								
3								
4								
5								
6								
7								
8								
9								

DOCUMENTATION OF NEW SCREENINGS AND EVALUATIONS
- Page 2 -

School Year: _____

Therapist: _____   School District: _____

Directions and codes: See previous page.

#	Last name	First name	School	Current grade	Referred by	Reason	Concern	Outcome
10								
11								
12								
13								
14								
15								
16								
17								
18								
19								
20								
21								
22								
23								
24								
25								

Note. GE = general education; IEP = individualized education program; OT = occupational therapy; SE = special education.

FORM 3.B. SAMPLE FORM FOR REQUEST FOR OCCUPATIONAL THERAPY SUPPORT—TEACHER

OCCUPATIONAL THERAPY DEPARTMENT
REQUEST FOR OCCUPATIONAL THERAPY SUPPORTS TO TEACHER

Note. All incomplete forms will be returned to individuals to complete.

Person Requesting Occupational Therapy Support: _____   Date: _____

School District: _____   Building: _____   Grade: _____

Contact: (phone) _____   (e-mail) _____

> Due to licensure laws in this state, occupational therapists cannot discuss specific students prior to a referral. General support such as "What can I use to help a student hold their pencil better" or "Look at this classroom work, and tell me if I should make a referral" are allowed. DO NOT SHARE ANY STUDENT OR FAMILY INFORMATION.

Reason you are requesting an occupational therapy support? (Describe the problem in terms of educational impact.)

_____

_____

_____

Please summarize your attempts to resolve this concern and results. (If applicable, attach classroom samples from target student and peers—remove names.)

_____

_____

_____

> Date completed form received by occupational therapist: _____
>
> Date occupational therapist initiated contact with requestor: _____

Notes:

_____

_____

_____

_____

_____

_____

FORM 3.C. SAMPLE FORM FOR REQUEST FOR OCCUPATIONAL THERAPY SUPPORT— CONSULTATION FOR STUDENT

OCCUPATIONAL THERAPY DEPARTMENT
REQUEST FOR OCCUPATIONAL THERAPY CONSULTATION FOR STUDENT

Note. All incomplete forms will be returned to individuals to complete.

Student's Name: _____   Date: _____

School District: _____   Building: _____   Grade: _____

Contact: Name: _____   (phone) _____   (e-mail) _____

Background Information:

• Student has passed vision screening: Yes ☐   No ☐

• Student has passed hearing screening: Yes ☐   No ☐

Has this concern been shared with others?

• Parents: Yes ☐   No ☐ (reason it was not shared) _____

• Building Team: Yes ☐   No ☐ (reason it was not shared) _____

Date parents were notified that you were contacting the occupational therapist for a general consultation? Date: _____
Response From Parent: Yes ☐   No ☐

Reason you are requesting occupational therapy support? (Describe the problem in terms of educational impact.)

_____

_____

_____

Please summarize your attempts to resolve this concern and results. (If applicable, attach classroom samples from target student and peers—remove names.)

_____

_____

_____

Please list any other areas of concerns being addressed by you or others. List any additional information that would be beneficial.

_____

_____

_____

OCCUPATIONAL THERAPY DEPARTMENT
REQUEST FOR OCCUPATIONAL THERAPY CONSULTATION FOR STUDENT
- Page 2 -

Date completed form received by occupational therapist: _____

Date occupational therapist initiated contact with requestor: _____

Notes:

_____

_____

_____

_____

_____

_____

_____

_____

_____

_____

_____

_____

_____

_____

_____

_____

_____

_____

_____

_____

FORM 3.D. QUESTIONS FOR INTERVIEWING PARENT AND TEACHER

INTERVIEW QUESTIONS

Student: _____ Person interviewed: _____ Date: _____

Directions: Complete one form for each person interviewed. Use the final column to check areas you want to further explore.

Questions—Encourage Specific Answers	Responses	Significant Yes or No
What is the student's current educational program, including any areas in which student is receiving assistance?		
What aspects of the educational program are going well, and what areas are not? (Be specific regarding supports or barriers in environment, instruction, curriculum, functional tasks.)		
What is the expected performance in the area of concern? (Note whether this is peer comparison, teacher expectation, building policy.)		
How is the student doing in other areas? (Give examples based on the student's age relating to ADLs, IADLs, rest and sleep, education, work, play, leisure, social participation.)		
What has been attempted to assist the student in this area of concern? Outcome of those attempts?		
Is this student frequently absent from school? Have any medical concerns? Pass visual and hearing screening?		
Other information pertinent to area of concern:		

Note. ADLs = activities of daily living; IADLs = instrumental activities of daily living.

FORM 3.E. QUESTIONS FOR INTERVIEWING STUDENTS

STUDENT INTERVIEW QUESTIONS

Student: _____   Date: _____

Questions—Encourage Specific Answers	Responses
What do you usually do after school? What do you usually do on weekends? Who do you like to spend time with? Tell me about your friends outside of school.	
What chores do you have at home? What do you do for fun?	
What do you like to do at school? What do you like learning about? What do you do at recess or when you have free time in the classroom? Who do you spend time with at school? Tell me about your friends at school.	
What things at school are frustrating? What things at school are you best at?	
Who is your favorite teacher? What does he or she do that helps you learn or have fun at school?	
What do you hope to learn in school this year? If your teacher let you choose anything to learn about, what would you choose?	
What would you like to do after you graduate from high school? What job would you like to have?	

FORM 3.F. DOCUMENTATION TEMPLATE USING RIOT

OCCUPATIONAL THERAPY
GENERAL EDUCATION: RIOT DOCUMENTATION

Student: _____ Birthdate: _____ Grade: _____

School: _____ Teacher: _____

INFORMAL SCREENING OF STUDENT'S OCCUPATIONS

Occupation	Any Concerns in This Area	Student's Performance	
		Successful	Problematic
ADLs—self-care (e.g., toileting, hygiene or grooming, dressing, eating, functional mobility, showering in PE)			
IADLs—home and community tasks (e.g., care of pets, community mobility, health management, meal preparation, safety)			
Rest and sleep (e.g., able to stay awake)			
Education (e.g., access, participation, academic and functional performance)			
Work (e.g., prevocational, volunteer, chores)			
Play and leisure (e.g., interests, opportunities, abilities)			
Social participation (e.g., interactions in community and with family and peers)			

R—RECORD REVIEW

Document information from medical and educational records that is significant at this time.

Student has passed recent vision screening: No ☐   Yes ☐

Student has passed recent hearing screening: No ☐   Yes ☐

Student has a known medical condition: No ☐   Yes ☐   List: _____

Student has been hospitalized or had surgery: No ☐   Yes ☐   List: _____

NOTES: _____

_____

OCCUPATIONAL THERAPY
GENERAL EDUCATION: RIOT DOCUMENTATION
- Page 2 -

Student: _____ Birthdate: _____ Grade: _____

I—INTERVIEW

General:

- Are student's language skills delayed?   No ☐   Yes ☐
- Does student have difficulty attending to tasks? No ☐   Yes ☐
- Does student have established hand preference?   No ☐   Yes ☐   List right or left: _____

1. Tell me about this student and things he or she does well (gather interests, talents).

2. How does the concern expressed earlier impact the student's educational program?

3. How long has this occurred?

4. Describe the expected performance in the natural environment. (What is expected performance based on?)

5. List activities, strategies, and modifications that you have tried and the results.

6. What are your priorities and hopes for this student?

7. Questions About Student and Environment	NO	YES	NOTES
• Safe and supportive school climate			
• Manages temporal context (i.e., routines, fatigue, rest)			
• Engages in social interactions during the day			
• Participates in educational program			
• Physically accesses building			
• Physically accesses classroom and equipment			
• Physically accesses bathrooms and equipment			
• Physically accesses playground or gym equipment			
• Physically accesses materials in school			
• Encourages independence (vs. adult dependence)			
• Access to school food, if applicable			
• Other			

OCCUPATIONAL THERAPY
GENERAL EDUCATION: RIOT DOCUMENTATION
- Page 3 -

Student: _____   Birthdate: _____   Grade: _____

Use the additional questions that are related to the concern(s):

Area	Question	NO	YES	NOTES
Self-Care	• Clothing fasteners			
	• Un/dressing			
	• Tying shoes			
	• PE dressing			
	• Toileting			
	• Washing hands			
	• Other			
	• Eating (if yes—see next questions)			
	• Student's current Ht _____ Wt _____ BMI _____			
	• Student's primary method of eating (orally, tube)			
	• Describe typical mealtime and student's performance			
	• Other			
Fine Motor	• Coloring			
	• Drawing			
	• Cutting			
	• Gluing			
	• Computer use			
	• Managing book bag			
	• Managing papers			
	• Lunchroom skills (e.g., using utensils)			
	• Other			

OCCUPATIONAL THERAPY
GENERAL EDUCATION: RIOT DOCUMENTATION
- Page 4 -

Student: _____ Birthdate: _____ Grade: _____

Use the additional questions that are related to the concern(s):

Area	Question	NO	YES	NOTES
Literacy	• Does the district have a specific handwriting curriculum that is taught with fidelity?			
	• How much time during the day is spent teaching handwriting?			
	• Does the student know all the names of the alphabet letters?			
	• Does the student know all of the sounds of the alphabet letters?			
	• Other			
Social Communication & Executive Functioning	• Does student appropriately indicate wants?			
	• Describe what student does if routines are changed?			
	• Does student take turns?			
	• How does student respond to frustration?			
	• Describe social interactions with peers. Adults?			
	• Describe student's level of play and leisure skills.			
	• Does student imitate?			
	• Does student sustain attention to the task?			
	• Does student display age-appropriate memory?			
	• Other			

OCCUPATIONAL THERAPY
GENERAL EDUCATION: RIOT DOCUMENTATION
- Page 5 -

Student: _____ Birthdate: _____ Grade: _____

O—OBSERVATION
FORM A

Setting and task observed:

Time	Task	Expected/Peer Performance	Target Student Performance	Comments

O—OBSERVATION
FORM B

Directions: Observe during the time the activity is to be performed. Check (✓) the last box if there are concerns in this area.

Setting:		
Activity:		
AREA	**Comments About Supports or Barriers in Each Area**	✓
Physical, sensory, and social environment		
Curriculum, instruction		
Motor skills		
Process skills		
Social interaction skills		
Mental, sensory, neuromusculo-skeletal functions		

OCCUPATIONAL THERAPY
GENERAL EDUCATION: RIOT DOCUMENTATION
- Page 6 -

Student: _____   Birthdate: _____   Grade: _____

T—TESTS/TOOLS

Test Administered	Date	Result

Notes:

_____

_____

_____

_____

_____

_____

_____

_____

_____

_____

Note. ADLs = activities of daily living; BMI = body mass index; Ht = height; IADLs = instrumental activities of daily living; PE = physical education; RIOT = review record, interview, observe, and test; Wt = weight.

FORM 3.G. OCCUPATIONAL PERFORMANCE OBSERVATIONS

OCCUPATIONAL PERFORMANCE OBSERVATIONS

Directions: Check the box to indicate the supports and skills observed. Under "Motor, Process, and Social Interaction Skills," circle or highlight the skills observed, and describe observations in the comment section.

Name: _____ Teacher: _____ Room: _____

Observation #1: _____ Date: _____ Time: _____

Observation #2: _____ Date: _____ Time: _____

Occupations[1] Observed

☐ ADLs (i.e., dressing, eating, functional mobility, personal device care, personal hygiene or grooming)

☐ IADLs (i.e, care of others, care of pets, communication management, driving and community mobility, financial management, meal preparation, safety and emergency maintenance, shopping)

☐ Rest and sleep (i.e, rest, sleep preparation and participation)

☐ Education (i.e., academic, nonacademic, extracurricular, vocational education, vocational interests)

☐ Social participation (i.e., community, family, peer or friend)

☐ Play (i.e., play exploration and participation)

☐ Leisure (i.e., leisure exploration and participation)

Context and Environment[1]

Environmental Supports	✓	Comments/Observations
Evidence-based classroom management strategies in place:[2] • Positive expectations for routines visible • Classroom provides adequate space and limited distractions • Transition signal provided (visual or auditory).		
Student's position in classroom supports attention and performance.		
Desk and chair height are appropriate for student.		
Physical environment is accessible.		
Social environment is supportive.		
Physical environment supports attention and performance (e.g., lighting, furniture, temperature, noises, activity level).		
Teacher Supports	✓	**Comments/Observations**
Evidence-based classroom management strategies in place:[1] • Prompts or precorrections are provided regarding expectations • Reinforcement is provided for following expectations • Feedback or correction provided for not following expectations.		
Clear instructions are provided for activity.		
Teacher expectations are appropriate.		
Feedback (visual or auditory) is provided regarding task performance or behavior.		

[1]AOTA (2014).
[2]Simonsen, Fairbanks, Briesch, Myers, & Sugai (2008).

Task Supports/Activity Demands	✓	Comments/Observations
Evidence-based classroom management strategies in place:[2]		
Task is engaging and interesting.		
Level of challenge is appropriate.		
Printed materials are clear and organized.		

Performance Patterns and Performance Skills[1]

Habits	✓	Comments/Observations
Demonstrates useful student habits.		
Demonstrates dominating or impoverished habits.		
Routines		
Understands and follows classroom routines.		
Has personal routines that support participation.		
Roles: Understands roles and meets roll expectations		
Motor Skills: Demonstrates adequate skills to meet activity demands		
Interacts with and moves task objects and self around environment: Aligns, stabilizes, positions, reaches, bends, grips, manipulates, coordinates, moves, lifts, walks, transports, calibrates, flows, endures, paces.		
Process Skills: Demonstrates adequate skill to meet activity demands		
Selects, interacts with and uses tools and materials, carries out individual actions and steps, modifies performance when problems are encountered: paces, attends, heeds, chooses, uses, handles, inquires, initiates, continues sequences, terminates, searches/locates, gathers, organizes, restores, navigates, notices and responds, adjusts, accommodates, benefits.		
Social Interaction Skills: Demonstrates adequate skills to meet activity demands		
Approaches or starts, concludes or disengages, produces speech, gesticulates, speaks fluently, turns toward, looks, places self, touches, regulates, questions, replies, discloses, expresses emotion, disagrees, thanks, transitions, times response, times duration, takes turns, matches language, clarifies, acknowledges and encourages, empathizes, heeds, accommodates, benefits.		
Comments/Recommendations		

---

[1]American Occupational Therapy Association. (2014). Occupational therapy practice framework: Domain and process (3rd ed.). *American Journal of Occupational Therapy, 68*(Suppl. 1), S1–S48. https://doi.org/10.5014/ajot.2014.682006

[2]Simonsen, B., Fairbanks, S., Briesch, A., Myers, D., & Sugai, G. (2008). Evidence-based practices in classroom management: Considerations for research to practice. *Education and Treatment of Children, 31*, 351–380.

FORM 3.H. SENSORY PROCESSING OBSERVATIONS

OBSERVATIONS OF SENSORY RESPONSES

Name: _____ Teacher: _____ Room: _____

Observation #1: _____ Date: _____ Time: _____

Observation #2: _____ Date: _____ Time: _____

SENSORY RESPONSES[1]

Sensory/Seeking	Sensory/Avoiding
Auditory, visual, light touch, deep pressure, movement, heavy work, proprioception, smell, taste, adult attention, oral–motor, peer attention	Auditory, visual, light touch, deep pressure, movement, heavy work, proprioception, smell, taste, adult attention, oral–motor, peer attention
Sensory/Sensitivity	**Low/Registration**
Auditory, visual, light touch, deep pressure, movement, heavy work, proprioception, smell, taste, adult attention, oral–motor, peer attention	Auditory, visual, light touch, deep pressure, movement, heavy work, proprioception, smell, taste, adult attention, oral–motor, peer attention

Comments/Recommendations:

[1]Dunn, W. (2014). *Sensory Profile–2.* Bloomington, MN: Psychological Corporation.

FORM 3.I. EXAMPLE OF A COMPLETED SENSORY PROCESSING OBSERVATIONS FORM

OBSERVATIONS OF SENSORY RESPONSES

Name: _____ Teacher: _____ Room: _____

SENSORY RESPONSES

Sensory/Seeking	Sensory/Avoiding
Auditory, visual, light touch, deep pressure, movement, heavy work, proprioception, **smell,** taste, adult attention, oral–motor, **peer attention** Jump, spin around, fidgeted with paper, made noises, smelled items (paper after coloring leaves), shock head, looked through hole in leaf using peripheral vision, waved items in peers face, chased peer, jiggled while standing in line	Auditory, visual, light touch, deep pressure, movement, heavy work, proprioception, smell, taste, adult attention, oral–motor, peer attention
Sensory/Sensitivity	Low/Registration
Auditory, visual, **light touch,** deep pressure, movement, heavy work, proprioception, smell, taste, adult attention, oral–motor, peer attention Showed student and moved away when bumped accidentally. Started crying and fell over when finger was accidentally stepped on.	**Auditory,** visual, **light touch,** deep pressure, movement, heavy work, proprioception, smell, taste, adult attention, oral–motor, peer attention Frequently needed multiple cues to respond to transition signals and other auditory cues. Did better when tracing with crayon vs. finger on tablet.

Comments/Recommendations:

- Appears to seek sensory input; may increased opportunities for movement.
- May be sensitive to and react aggressively or emotionally to unexpected touch. Try positioning at back of group or provide designated space where bumping is likely.
- May be slow to process and respond to auditory cues; may need cues to be enhanced (e.g., use visual and auditory cues, provide "warning" prior to giving cue).
- Decreased responsiveness to verbal directions was observed in English-language class, so language barrier may be a factor. Difficulty processing and responding to auditory input may make learning second language more difficult.

FORM 3.J. GATHERING ABC DATA

Student: _____ Birthdate: _____ Date: _____

Environment (Where?)	Antecedent (What happened?)	Behavior (What was student's response?)	Consequence (What happened?)

Notes:

_____

_____

_____

_____

_____

_____

_____

_____

_____

_____

_____

_____

_____

FORM 3.K. SAMPLE OF ABC DATA

Environment (Where?)	Antecedent (What happened?)	Behavior (What was student's response?	Consequence (What happened?)
In the hallway	Peer accidently bumps into Mason	Mason hits peer in the arm	Teacher aware that Mason is very sensitive to people in his space/touching him and reacts with anger/frustration. Teacher had students apologize to each other and contacted the parents to let them know this was an accidental and reflexive interaction.

Notes: Mason had an occupational therapy evaluation a few months ago, and the teacher was given information about children with sensory processing disorders, especially tactile hypersensitivity. This increased the teacher's awareness of how to handle this encounter.

FORM 3.L. SAMPLE OF AN OCCUPATIONAL THERAPY REPORT TEMPLATE

OCCUPATIONAL THERAPY REPORT TEMPLATE

Name: _____ Birthdate: _____ Grade: _____
Parents: _____ Phone: _____
Address: _____
School district: _____ School building: _____
Report written by: _____ Date: _____
Medical conditions: _____

Referral information: Indicate who made the referral and why. Also list any information about general education activities, if appropriate.

Occupational profile: Include current occupations in the least restrictive environment that are successful and that are problematic. When possible, list peers' performance to demonstrate the need for services. List any significant medical, education, or work history. List parent, teacher, and student priorities and targeted outcomes.

Assessments used and results: Identify gathered information. List any assessments used and their results (including interviews, observations, standardized assessments, and nonstandardized assessments). List peers' performance on the task.

Summary and analysis: Discuss and summarize data as they relate to the student's occupational profile and referring concern. Delineate the specific area(s) of occupation on which intervention will focus. List instructional needs, including modifications and accommodations. Make judgment regarding appropriateness of occupational therapy services or suggest other services.

FORM 3.M. SAMPLE EVALUATION REPORT

OCCUPATIONAL THERAPY REPORT—CONFIDENTIAL INFORMATION REMOVED

Name: <u>Noah J.</u>   Birthdate: _____   Grade: _____

Parents: _____   Phone: _____

Address: _____

Attending district: _____   Attending building: _____

Occupational therapist: _____   Date: _____

Medical conditions: <u>autism spectrum disorder (ASD), attention deficit/hyperactivity disorder (ADHD), low muscle tone.</u>

Referral information:

Due to Noah's academic and motor skills, his first-grade general education (GE) teacher had contacted the parents, Building Assistance Team, and the district occupational therapist. GE interventions (supplemental and intensive assistance) were provided for 7 weeks, but minimal changes were noted. Last year he struggled, but parents felt he would catch up if given more time. His father consented to a full and individual initial evaluation for academics as well as occupational therapy.

Occupational profile:

The following information was gathered from his father and teacher. Noah lives with his father, stepmother, and younger sibling. Biological mother died last year. He was born full term and met milestones until age 2. Skills were slow to develop at that time, and some regression was noted. He was diagnosed with ADHD first, then ASD. Very slow weight gain, so medications for ADHD have been changed to improve diet. Attendance is good (missed 2 days due to illness).

OCCUPATIONS	SUMMARY OF PERFORMANCE WITHIN THE EDUCATIONAL PROGRAM AND ACTIVITIES
Activities of daily living	Independent in toileting and eating. Unable to zip jeans, un/button small buttons on coat, or tie shoes. Generally, he wears pull-over shirts. Takes a long time to eat and gags on some textures of food (e.g. mashed potatoes, catsup).
Rest and sleep	No concern expressed by parent in this area; not sleepy at school.
Education	Need modifications and adult physical assistance to complete written work and fine motor skills. Easily distracted.
Work	Not applicable (has chores at home).
Play and leisure	Frustrated because he breaks toys easily and does not have motor skills (e.g., balance, strength) to keep up with peers on playground.
Social participation	Difficulty with peer interactions. Easily frustrated, cries, and screams.

Assessments used and results:

Noah was cooperative during the evaluation, which was conducted using record review of medical status, interview, observation, and a standardized test. Information from school records is listed below.

OCCUPATIONAL THERAPY REPORT—CONFIDENTIAL INFORMATION REMOVED
- Page 2 -

Name: Noah J. _____ Birthdate: _____ Grade: _____

DATE	METHODS USED	RESULTS
1/3/17	**Interview**	See table in previous section.
1/10/17	**Observation of** Self-care	Noah tangled up his coat when attempting to put it on. Adult assistance needed to untangle. Used flip-over method (other peers put on coat using typical method). Asked paraprofessional for help with zipper before trying it on his own. He noticed his shoe was not tied but did not request help or attempt to tie it.
	Recess and social interaction	Noah attempted to play soccer game with peers. He can kick ball if it is still and made attempts to keep up with peers when running, but he struggled. He fell 4 times (none of the peers fell). On playground equipment, he had to hold rail to ascend the stairs. Fell on movable walk area, crying, and needed assistance to get off.
	Fine motor activities	Great ideas but lacks sound–letter skills, so unable to write words. Always starts an activity but doesn't complete. Very cooperative. While classroom peers were using tools independently and completing tasks, Noah could not position them correctly in his hand or use them without moderate to maximum assistance.
1/10/17	**Tools** Automatic letter writing and numbers	From dictation and out of sequence, Noah correctly formed 7:26 capital letters (27% accurate); 7:26 lowercase letters (27% accurate). (Primarily letters in his name.) Writing numbers 1–8 in order resulted in 2:8 (25%) accuracy. Typical classroom peers could correctly form over 90% of upper and lower letters and numbers.
	Journal writing	Noah's samples were compared to 3 classroom peers. He typically wrote 2 words (9 letters) and stopped. None of the letters (0%) were legible due to light pressure, poor formation, and irregular spacing. Peers wrote 4–8 words (201 letters) that were over 90% legible.
	Developmental Test of Visual Perception–2	This standardized assessment tool provides information on visual perception (e.g., finding the same design) and visual–motor integration (e.g., using pencil to copy paths, dots, or pictures). Noah's scores were below the 5th percentile (very low). Form constancy (picking the same form even though it was bigger, smaller, darker, or oriented different than the model) was his strength (within average). Other areas, such as connecting dots with a straight line or tracing on a line, were very low.

Summary and Analysis:

Occupational performance: Noah demonstrates strengths in his ability to initiate tasks, seek help when necessary, and have great ideas. Participation in the fine motor classroom activities is discrepant from peers. He is unable to perform most of the fine motor skills in the classroom without adult assistance (to stay on task, to finish task, to complete task). Social interactions and playground activities are barriers to his educational performance. The IEP team should consider occupational therapy services for Noah to enhance participation.

Educational needs: The following describes Noah's educational needs in order for him to benefit from his educational program:

- *Instruction:* Noah is easily distracted when working in the classroom. Providing him with an additional "work" area with less distraction enhanced his ability to work with 25% less adult prompting. Providing easy tasks first to build his confidence motivated him to attempt more complex tasks.
- *Curriculum:* Noah needs to learn letter and number formation so he can form them automatically. He needs to learn spacing and placement on a line. Developing dexterity (in-hand manipulation) in his fingers should enhance fine motor coordination and tool use (e.g., pencil, scissors, crayons). Self-care skills (e.g., putting on coat, tying shoes) must be practiced to gain independence. Large motor endurance, balance, and upper-body strength must be developed to enhance playground and social interaction skills. Assistive technology for writing should be considered for next year if he is struggling with written language.
- *Environment:* Noah does not work well in noisy environments (e.g., busy hallway, cafeteria, classroom). Placement near the edges of the room would lessen the noises. Modifying area for less visual and auditory distractions would benefit him.

_____
Occupational therapist signature

FORM 3.N. SAMPLE REEVALUATION REPORT

OCCUPATIONAL THERAPY REEVALUATION REPORT—CONFIDENTIAL INFORMATION REMOVED

Name: <u>Lettie J.</u>_____ Birthdate: _____ Grade: 3 _____

Parents: _____ Phone: _____

Address: _____

School district: _____ School building: _____

Report written by: _____ Date: _____

Evaluation purpose and methods:

An occupational therapy evaluation was completed as part of a special education (SE) 3-year reevaluation. The purpose of the evaluation was to help determine continued eligibility for special education and identify student strengths and needs, including SE services and supports. Evaluation included record review, analysis of occupational performance during structured activities and in the classroom, teacher and staff interview, and standardized assessments as follows:

- Beery–Buktenica Developmental Test of Visual–Motor Integration, 6th Edition (VMI–6), a standardized, norm-referenced test that measures how well visual perception works together with finger and hand movements and includes 2 supplemental tests that measure visual discrimination/perception and motor coordination.

- School Function Assessment (SFA), a criterion-referenced, standardized assessment of school performance based on observations of the student within the school setting and on the judgment of the teachers and other school staff who work with the child; 95% of children score at or above criterion on this test.

- Sensory Profile 2, a set of standardized, judgment-based caregiver and teacher questionnaires designed to measure a child's sensory processing patterns and determine how sensory processing may be influencing participation.

Record review:

Lettie began receiving early intervention services as a toddler. She was enrolled in a developmental preschool program at age 3 and received a medical diagnosis of autism at age 4. She was last evaluated by occupational therapy as a kindergartner. At that time, she demonstrated a significant delay (2.0 *SD*) on the fine motor subtests of the Peabody Developmental Motor Scales. Although Lettie demonstrated functional abilities in some areas that were not represented in the test scores, she demonstrated delays in fine motor and specially designed instruction in the area of fine motor skills was recommended with occupational therapy provided as a related service.

Behavior during testing:

Lettie transitioned readily to testing. She was generally cooperative, but her performance was variable depending on her interest in and attention to the activity. Her verbal interactions were limited. She was slow to respond to direct questions and benefited from visual supports such as picture communication symbols. Lettie had difficulty maintaining visual attention and following verbal directions during structured standardized assessment and did better when directions were modeled. Evaluation procedures were valid and results are considered to be a reliable measure of her functional performance, although her visual perception skills may be higher than VMI–6 test scores indicate.

Occupational performance observations:

- *Recess:* Lettie went directly to the fence at the front of the playground. She played by herself, either standing and watching the cars or running back and forth along the fence. Other girls from her class played together and used playground equipment.
- *PE:* Lettie participated in several games that involved catching, kicking, and throwing at a target. She followed the rules with moderate assistance and was able to kick, throw, and catch similarly to her peers. She had difficulty maintaining attention throughout each game but participated well when the activity interested her.
- *Writer's workshop:* Lettie needed assistance to use the mouse to create a picture on the computer. She had difficulty coordinating her mouse clicks and tended to click and drag with the mouse rather than clicking to select the stamp she wanted. Other students in the class were able to create pictures independently. She had no difficulty using the mouse to make scribbles, and she seemed to enjoy this activity. When typing, she pressed 1 letter key and held it down to create long strings of repeated letters. She tired of the activity after about 5 minutes and requested a break with prompting. The other students remained on task for 15–20 minutes.

OCCUPATIONAL THERAPY REEVALUATION REPORT—CONFIDENTIAL INFORMATION REMOVED
- Page 2 -

Name: Lettie J.   Birthdate: _____   Grade: 3

Occupational profile:
- *Strengths and interests:* Lettie enjoys looking at books, putting puzzles together, and playing with therapy putty. She likes Dora the Explorer and playing hide and seek.
- *Group participation:* Lettie participates in a weekly fine motor group with 3 of her classmates. She transitions appropriately when given a visual schedule and a transition picture. She does not follow directions given to the group and needs multiple, individually directed cues to initiate each step of a multistep project.
- *Arts and crafts activities:* When focused, Lettie accurately completes fine motor tasks such as cutting shapes, coloring, writing her name, and using the glue stick with minimal assistance. She draws recognizable pictures and orients shapes appropriately when given a model to copy.
- *Handwriting:* Lettie wrote all of the letters of the alphabet from memory with 22/26 uppercase and 21/26 lowercase letters legible (i.e., letters could be identified as the intended letter). Having a model to copy did not improve legibility. Lettie's performance for both copying and writing letters from memory was inconsistent. She wrote 4 out of 52 letters within the lines of 3/8" wide 3-line paper. The rest of the letters varied in size from about 3\4" to 1 3\4". She briefly used a tripod grasp when given a pencil grip and assistance to position her fingers but quickly reverted to a whole-hand grasp. She is easily frustrated during handwriting lessons in the classroom and requires frequent breaks and clear expectations (including what she is expected to do, how much work needs to be completed, and what activity is next) to support attention and compliance.
- *Writing:* During writing lessons, Lettie is often reluctant to write and has difficulty generating her own ideas. She has typed several words when given direct cuing and a model to copy. When asked to write independently on a self-selected topic at the computer, Lettie types strings of letters with no spaces or identifiable words. However, when given the opportunity to draw freely, she drew a horse and wrote the word "horse."
- *Activities of daily living:* Lettie is not yet toilet trained. She follows a toileting schedule. She has difficulty with clothing fasteners, including buttons and separating zippers. When washing her hands, she rinses the soap off without rubbing her hands together. At lunch she uses utensils appropriately and opens packages independently.
- *Priorities and outcomes:* Lettie's teacher reported that her priorities for Lettie for the coming year included behavior management, following school-related self-care routines, handling transitions, and participating in writing activities. Lettie's mother had similar concerns regarding handling transitions, regulating behavior, and following self-care routines at home. She would also like Lettie to interact more with her classmates.

Assessment results:
- *Visual–motor and visual–perceptual skills:* The VMI–6 was used to determine if difficulties with visual–motor skills was affecting handwriting performance. Lettie demonstrated significant delays for her age (below the 1st percentile, 2.0 *SD* below the mean) on the visual–motor (form copying) section of this test and on the supplemental motor coordination test. Although she also demonstrated significant delays in the area of visual perception (1st percentile, 2.0 *SD* below the mean), visual perception appears to be an area of strength, and her actual abilities may be higher than test scores indicate. She often identified the correct shape, recognizing subtle differences despite responding impulsively without taking time to carefully review each option, and she had several correct responses after three consecutive failures.

- *Sensory processing:* The Sensory Profile 2, School Companion, was completed by Lettie's teacher and was used to identify Lettie's general patterns of behavioral responses to different types of sensory input. The patterns of behavior are divided into 4 quadrants: Seeking/Seeker, Avoiding/Avoider, Sensitivity/Sensor, and Registration/Bystander. On this assessment, Lettie demonstrated sensory processing challenges in all areas. Her scores on this assessment were as follows:
  - *Seeking/Seeker* represents the extent to which the student enjoys highly stimulating sensory environments, creates sensory input for herself, and has difficulty tolerating environments that offer limited sensory experiences. Lettie scored in the "more than others" range in this area, indicating that she may create additional sensory input for herself through visual input (watching fast-moving images or brightly colored graphics on the computer), touch (e.g., touching objects, textures, and people), movement activities (e.g., fidgeting with objects, running), and oral–motor input (chewing on nonfood items). Through sensory seeking, she may be trying to give herself the input she needs to stay alert at school.
  - *Avoiding/Avoider* represents the extent to which the student purposefully withdraws from or limits sensory input, tries to make sensations in the environment more predictable, and becomes overwhelmed when there is a higher level of sensory stimulation in the environment. Lettie scored at the "much more than others" level in this area. While she seeks movement input, she is slower to participate in physically active tasks compared to her peers, and she refuses to participate in team games. She also tends to be inflexible and is distressed when there are changes in routine. She avoids participating in group activities, suggesting that she may need time to prepare herself for movement activities, especially when they are not self-selected and predictable.
  - *Sensitivity/Sensor* represents the extent to which the student readily responds to sensations, perceives sensations that other people aren't aware of, are highly attentive to sensations in the environment, or are easily distracted. Lettie scored as "more than others" in this area. She appears to be more sensitive to auditory input (e.g., loud noises, fire alarms, and group activities where there is a lot of talking) than other students. She is sometimes bothered by touch input (such as when her hands are messy) and during movement activities that are not self-selected and predictable such as when standing or walking in a line with others.
  - *Registration/Bystander* represents the extent to which the student misses sensations that are present in the environment, underreacts or is slow to react to sensory input, and is able to attend when there are distractions in the environment. Lettie scored as "much more than others" in this area. While she may be sensitive to loud noises, she is slow to respond to verbal directions. She also misses demonstrated directions, struggles to keep her materials organized, and skips items on a busy worksheet.

- *School participation and performance:* The SFA was used to help identify Lettie's strengths and limitations in functional, nonacademic school tasks that may be affecting school participation. The assessment is divided into 3 areas: Participation, Task Supports, and Activity Performance. The 3 areas were rated by Lettie's SE classroom teacher and compared to peers in her highly structured, self-contained SE classroom.

OCCUPATIONAL THERAPY REEVALUATION REPORT—CONFIDENTIAL INFORMATION REMOVED
- Page 3 -

Name: Lettie J.   Birthdate: _____   Grade: 3

1. *Participation.* This section measured Lettie's level of participation in 6 major school settings. Her criterion score was 55, which is below the criterion cutoff for her grade/placement (criterion cutoff = 100). Her scores in the area of participation were

- SE class – 3 *(participation in all aspects with constant supervision)*
- Playground/recess – 2 *(participation in a few activities)*
- Transportation – 4 *(participation in all aspects with occasional assistance)*
- Bathroom/toileting – 3 *(participation in all aspects with constant supervision)*
- Transitions – 4 *(participation in all aspects with occasional assistance)*
- Mealtime/snack time – 5 *(modified full participation).*

2. *Task Supports.* This section measured the level of assistance (adult help) and adaptations (e.g., modifications to equipment, environment, or activity) that are needed to support performance in physical tasks and cognitive/behavioral tasks at school. The level of assistance and adaptations provided for the 9 physical task areas was rated as follows:

	PHYSICAL TASKS—ASSISTANCE	PHYSICAL TASKS—ADAPTATIONS
None	Maintaining and changing positions	Travel, maintaining and changing positions, eating and drinking, and clothing management
Minimal	Travel, recreational movement, manipulation with movement (e.g., carrying materials, opening doors, retrieving items), eating and drinking, and clothing management	Recreational movement and manipulation with movement
Moderate	Using materials, setup and cleanup, and hygiene	Using materials, setup and cleanup, and hygiene
	COGNITIVE/BEHAVIORAL TASKS—ASSISTANCE	COGNITIVE/BEHAVIORAL TASKS—ADAPTATIONS
Minimal	None	Functional communication, and memory and understanding
Moderate	Functional communication, memory and understanding, following social conventions, compliance with adult directives and school rules, task behavior and completion, positive interaction, behavior regulation, personal care awareness, and safety	Following social conventions, compliance with adult directives and school rules, task behavior and completion, positive interaction, behavior regulation, personal care awareness, and safety

Lettie's classroom is highly structured and provides a high level of adaptations and support for all students. Adaptations in place for Lettie at the time of the assessment included

- Lettie wears a diaper and is on a toileting schedule.
- Lettie has a quiet area in the reading nook she uses as a calm-down space.
- Lettie has a visual schedule and is given frequent breaks and reinforcers. She is given extended time for activities as well as frequent feedback and monitoring.
- Lettie uses a pencil with a pencil grip and modified writing paper.
- Lettie requires an alternative curriculum and adjusted expectations for all academic subject areas. Opportunities for additional repetition and practice are included in her schedule. Directions are modified with visual supports, demonstrations, and modeling.

3. *Activity Performance.* The Physical Activity Performance scale measured Lettie's performance in school-related physical tasks and cognitive/behavioral tasks. In general, Lettie demonstrates strengths in the area of physical task performance and weaknesses in the area of cognitive/behavioral tasks. Her physical task criterion scores ranged from 48 to 92. She scored significantly below criterion in 10 of 11 physical task areas and less than 2 SE scores below criterion in 1 area (maintaining and changing positions). Going up and down stairs was not measured because there are no stairs at the school. In the area of cognitive/behavioral tasks, Lettie's criterion scores ranged from 40–57. She scored significantly below criterion in all 9 cognitive/behavioral task areas. Her criterion scores were as follows:

OCCUPATIONAL THERAPY REEVALUATION REPORT—CONFIDENTIAL INFORMATION REMOVED
- Page 4 -

Name: Lettie J.   Birthdate: _____   Grade: 3

PHYSICAL TASKS	CRITERION SCORE	CRITERION* CUTOFF	COGNITIVE/BEHAVIORAL TASKS	CRITERION SCORE	CRITERION CUTOFF
Travel	73	100	Functional communication	46	91
Maintaining and changing positions	92	100	Memory and understanding	51	79
Recreational movement	65	83	Following social conventions	47	73
Manipulation with movement	76	93	Compliance with adult directives and school rules	50	76
Using materials	63	83	Task behavior/completion	47	72
Setup and cleanup	67	87	Positive interaction	51	81
Eating and drinking	76	100	Behavior regulation	46	74
Hygiene	56	92	Personal care awareness	57	92
Clothing management	72	93	Safety	40	91
Up and down stairs	NA	100			
Written work	48	73			
Computer and equipment use	55	65	*95% of children score at or above the criterion cutoff score.		

- *Physical task strengths.* Lettie consistently changes positions as required during the day and gets in and out of the car independently. She moves throughout the classroom and school grounds, including moving on uneven surfaces. Lettie plays on a scooter board and on the climbing structure on the playground. She throws and catches a large ball consistently. Lettie uses a stapler, molds and shapes clay, paints with a brush, and cuts out simple shapes. She opens and closes a variety of containers, including milk cartons, and sealed bags. Lettie drinks from a cup without spilling and drinks from a water fountain. She typically brings finger foods for lunch, but when given an opportunity to use utensils, she demonstrated scooping food with a spoon and a fork and spearing food with a fork. Lettie puts on and removes clothing independently. She writes her first name with reasonable legibility and can type her first and last name.

- *Physical task areas of difficulty.* Lettie demonstrated inconsistent performance in many physical tasks compared to her peers, but her greatest areas of difficulty were in the areas of hygiene, written work, and computer and equipment use. Lettie wears a pull-up diaper and needs significant cueing to follow self-care routines, including washing her hands, caring for her toileting needs, wiping her face and hands, and blowing her nose. She has difficulty with most writing tasks, including identifying where to start and stop on a writing paper or worksheet, sizing her letters appropriately, and spacing between words. She has difficulty using a computer mouse and needs significant cueing to locate and hit 2 or more keys in sequence (e.g., control–alt–delete to log on). This limits her ability to access computer-based learning activities and specialized software supports available in her classroom. Other areas of difficulty include understanding and following game rules; cutting off tape from a tape dispenser; inserting a paper into a folder pocket; using a paper clip; passing out and collecting materials from her classmates; and manipulating clothing fasteners, including securing her shoes, separating and hooking a zipper, and buttoning a row of buttons.

- *Cognitive/behavioral task strengths.* Lettie usually demonstrates understanding directions, including basic 1-step directions, directions that involve conditional or sequential concepts (e.g., if/then), and directions involving prepositions or spatial concepts. She frequently acknowledges when someone says "thank you" and, given a prompt, will use good manners such as saying "please" or "sorry." Given a prompt, Lettie helps with cleanup tasks and follows rules regarding movement around the classroom and school. She consistently attends to audio/visual presentations for at least 20 minutes. Given a prompt, Lettie responds appropriately to social interactions from adults and peers. With minimal prompting, she maintains behavioral control during assemblies. Lettie consistently communicates yes/no, choices between 2 or more items, and her first and last name. She also communicates hungry/thirsty, sick/hurt/help, and where something is located in the classroom or school given minimal prompting.

- *Cognitive/behavioral task areas of difficulty.* Although Lettie demonstrated inconsistent performance on many cognitive/behavioral tasks compared to her peers, her greatest areas of difficulty were in the areas of functional communication, behavior regulation, personal care awareness, and safety. Lettie has difficulty communicating short messages, requesting information, and describing objects. She does not communicate what she would do if lost or other basic safety information. Lettie demonstrates self-stimulation by wiggling her fingers in front of her eyes, and she often disengages from school activities by repeating scripts from favorite cartoons to herself. She has difficulty accepting changes in routine and handling frustration. Transitions from preferred to nonpreferred activities are often difficult and may result in throwing items or running to the pillows in the reading area. Lettie needs reminders to initiate most personal care tasks, including wiping her face, washing and drying hands, wiping herself and redressing after toileting, wiping her nose, and closing the bathroom door for privacy. She needs constant supervision to support safety, including using caution around electrical equipment, items that are hot, and in situations where falling is possible; following the emergency exit routine; keeping unsafe objects out of her mouth; and safely crossing traffic areas. Other areas of difficulty include following 2- or 3-step directions, maintaining appropriate social/physical boundaries, asking for permission, waiting for her turn, sharing materials, and cooperating with nonroutine tasks. She has difficulty recovering after failure and withdraws rather than asking for help when directions are unclear.

OCCUPATIONAL THERAPY REEVALUATION REPORT—CONFIDENTIAL INFORMATION REMOVED
- Page 5 -

Name: Lettie J. _____ Birthdate: _____ Grade: 3_____

Summary and analysis:

Lettie is a sweet and playful girl with a diagnosis of ASD. Based on this evaluation, Lettie continues to demonstrate difficulties with occupational performance within the school environment. On the SFA, she demonstrated significant weaknesses with physical tasks, especially in the areas of hygiene, written work, and computer and equipment use. Lettie also demonstrated significant difficulties with many cognitive/behavioral tasks, supporting the need for specially designed instruction in the areas of adaptive skills and social/emotional/behavioral skills. In the area of visual–motor skills, Lettie demonstrated difficulties with pencil grasp and fine motor coordination for handwriting and for effectively using the computer. She also demonstrated sensory processing challenges, which may affect her ability to register and respond to sensory information within the school environment.

Factors that support Lettie's participation at school:
- Lettie demonstrates multiple interests within the school environment. She explores movement activities and loves looking at books.
- Lettie attempts challenging activities when given support and structure.
- Lettie is aware of daily classroom routines and cooperates with routine activities given support and redirection.
- Lettie accesses the school campus and participates in movement activities, including running, ball skills, and playing on movable play equipment.
- Lettie uses many tools and materials effectively, including scissors, staplers, erasers, and pencil sharpeners.

Lettie is currently placed in a self-contained SE classroom where she receives a high level of environmental supports, including
- School environment provides predictable school routines and a low student-to-teacher ratio.
- Classwork and expectations are modified to meet Lettie's learning needs.
- A quiet reading area is available for break time.
- Social environment is positive and supportive.

Specific areas of challenge for Lettie include
- Lettie needs multiple cues and significant support to perform activities associated with her toileting routine.
- Lettie is aware of activities associated with being a student but needs multiple cues and support to engage productively in classroom learning activities.
- Lettie has difficulty interacting and cooperating with others and sharing materials. She plays by herself at recess.
- Lettie has difficulty adapting her responses to solve problems and often gets frustrated or avoids difficult activities.
- Lettie has difficulty with maintaining an appropriate pencil grasp and engaging in writing activities. Grasp may be affected by low registration of touch input and/or limited hand strength.
- Lettie demonstrates sensory processing challenges in all areas.

GE impact: Lettie's sensory processing challenges, difficulties with performing many functional school tasks, and difficulties with hand coordination and pencil grasp affect her ability to engage in adult-directed learning activities, interact with peers, and access writing activities at school. Compared to her same-age peer without disabilities, Lettie needs increased predictability, teacher guidance, and supervision as well as modifications and sensory-based strategies to support behavior regulation, social interaction, and participation in school activities.

Recommendations:
- Provide support for developing increased independence in adaptive and social–emotional–behavioral skills. Lettie may need visual supports as well as direct instruction to learn hygiene routines and social interaction skills.
- Work on developing a more mature pencil grasp, including using an adapted pencil/pencil grip and developing hand skills. This will support handwriting fluency.
- Work on developing mouse skills at the computer. This will help Lettie access computer-based learning activities and assistive technology to support writing activities.
- Explore sensory-based strategies to support behavior regulation and school participation. Once successful strategies have been identified, they can be incorporated into Lettie's daily program. The following sensory strategies may be helpful for Lettie:
    - Provide high-interest visual input (e.g., bright colors and visually interesting activities).
    - Offer utensils that have a variety of textures or added weight.
    - Provide hand fidgets and oral–motor tools.
    - Schedule whole-class stretch or movement breaks.
    - Give Lettie jobs that require movement, such as passing out or collecting materials.
    - Establish predictable daily routines and incorporate repetition and predictability during movement activities and group time.
    - Provide visual supports to go along with verbal information.
    - Offer breaks in a quiet area of the classroom.
- Occupational therapy is recommended as a related service to support social–emotional–behavioral, adaptive, and written language goals. Occupational therapy services will include both hands-on services and team supports to develop hand strength and hand skills for pencil grasp, to improve mouse skills to support access to computer-based learning activities, to support social interaction, and to adapt activities to support successful participation as well as supporting ongoing problem solving related to sensory-based accommodations and supports. As Lettie's functional participation improves and she is able to regulate her behavior, interact with peers, access written-language activities, and follow school-related self-care routines, it is anticipated that occupational therapy will be discontinued unless additional needs are identified by the individualized education program team.

_____
Occupational therapist signature

Intervention: Planning, Implementation, and Review

4

Occupational therapy intervention consists of three phases: (1) planning, (2) implementation, and (3) review (American Occupational Therapy Association [AOTA], 2014). In the school setting, the education team's determination that a student has a disability and needs special education (SE) and related services initiates the intervention planning phase by developing that student's individualized education program (IEP). On the basis of the results of the student's free and individual evaluation, the team may identify occupational therapy as one of the related services needed for the student to benefit from his or her educational program. (*Note.* Some states allow occupational therapy to be considered "special education services" or "support services" and be the only SE service the student has on his or her IEP).

Table 4.1 lists some of the different forms identified under the Individuals with Disabilities Education Improvement Act of 2004 (IDEA; P. L. 108–446) that an occupational therapy practitioner may help complete during intervention planning, implementation, and review. Each state has documentation requirements based on the state's interpretation and implementation of IDEA. The forms and procedures used to document a student's IEP and other IDEA requirements are determined by the local school district and must comply with state and federal regulations.

DEVELOPING IEP GOALS

Using the evaluation reports from various professions, the IEP team members are responsible for developing the student's IEP, including the

Table 4.1. FORMS REQUIRED UNDER IDEA FOR THE INTERVENTION PROCESS

FORM AND IDEA REFERENCE	PURPOSE
IEP (34 CFR §300.321)	Documents the student's strengths and needs, current performance, and decisions made by the IEP team, including the student's proposed or current educational program, such as annual goals, services, modifications and supports, and participation with children without disabilities.
Parent consent for services (34 CFR §300.300[b])	Documents parents' consent to allow the provision of special education and related services for their child; also used for parental consent for additional evaluations or any changes in services and programs.
Progress reports to family	Provides parents with a description of how their child is progressing toward achieving annual IEP goals.
Transition plan (for students age 16 years at the time of the IEP or who meet the state transition age; 34 CFR §300.320[b])	Describes the student's postsecondary goals and the services needed to support goal achievement.
Summary of performance (34 CFR §300.305[e])	Provides a summary of the child's academic achievement and functional performance, including recommendations for assisting the child with meeting postsecondary goals; must be provided when students are no longer eligible for services because of age or graduation.

Note. IDEA = Individuals with Disabilities Education Improvement Act of 2004; IEP = individualized education program.

student's goals. These goals should be based on the student's strengths and needs, the student's current level of performance, and team priorities. A four-step approach to developing goals is outlined in Table 4.2. The table provides the example of Jill, a junior high student who enjoys picking out clothing and wearing a blue color streak in her hair. Jill had several peers she used to hang out with at school, but lately they have not been wanting to hang around. When she mentioned that to her SE teacher, the teacher stated that Jill has very bad breath. Because of physical and intellectual limitations, she is unable to brush her teeth, so her mother had been doing that for her. However, her mother's job now requires her to be at work earlier, so Jill

has been coming to school without her teeth brushed. The occupational therapist was contacted to help with this area.

DETERMINING RANGE OF SERVICE

The *Occupational Therapy Practice Framework: Domain and Process* (AOTA, 2014) lists the types of interventions and therapy approaches occupational therapists use. If occupational therapy services are determined to be necessary by the IEP team (including the occupational therapist), the occupational therapist typically recommends the amount and frequency, or range, of service.

Table 4.2. FOUR-STEP APPROACH TO STUDENT GOAL WRITING

STEP	EXAMPLE
1. Gather information through the occupational profile (through collaboration with teachers and family to establish the area of concern, baseline, and expected performance).	The teacher would like **Jill**, a junior high student, to perform daily life activities independently. Jill has a right hemiplegia and moderate intellectual impairment. She is unable to brush her teeth. The bad odor affects her relationships with peers.
2. Define the desired performance.	(What?) Jill will put toothpaste onto her toothbrush and brush her teeth.
3. Identify the conditions.	(When?) By 3-9-17. (Where?) In the girls' bathroom after lunch (other conditions), with an adult present.
4. Establish the criterion.	(How will we know it is met?) Jill will complete this task independently for 3 out of 5 consecutive days.

Completed goal: By 3-9-17, in girls' bathroom after lunch and with an adult present, Jill will put toothpaste onto her toothbrush and brush her teeth independently for 3 out of 5 consecutive days.

Note. Adapted from Frolek Clark (2013). Adapted with permission.

Table 4.3. EXAMPLE OF A RANGE OF SERVICE PLAN

RANGE OF SERVICE SUGGESTED	1	2	3	4
Occupational therapy services	15–30 min/quarter			180–240 min/mo

The range of service guidelines (see Form 4.A, "Range of Service Guidelines"), which scores 5 factors from 1 to 4, was designed to assist practitioners in making those decisions.

There are two parts to determining range of service. Part one is for the occupational therapy department to complete the range of service table (see Table 4.3 and bottom of table in Form 4.A). To do so, the department should determine the range of service within its boundaries. For instance, the department may decide that for a student with an IEP who meets all of the criteria listed in the "4" column of Form 4.A, range of service should be 45–60 min/wk, or 180–240 min/mo. Therefore, this range is entered under the "4" at the bottom of Form 4.A; see Table 4.3). For the student who has received intensive services and now scores a 1 on Form 4.A, he or she is determined to require 15–30 min/quarter of service, and this range is entered under the "1" at the bottom of Form 4.A (see Table 4.3). The department should determine range of service for each score in Form 4.A.

Part two in determining the range of service is to ascertain the median score for factors in Form 4.A for the student being suggested for occupational therapy services (or whose program is being reviewed). The median (middle) score is used because it disregards the outliers (e.g., 1, 4, 4, 3, 4; median is 4) and is a better indicator of the student's needs. After the therapist has read each factor and scored it (1–4; no fractions, e.g., 2.5, are allowed), the next step is to calculate the median score. Using this

score, the therapist would determine the appropriate range of service. Note that the therapist's professional judgment should always be considered when determining range of service, regardless of median score. For example, a student whose factor scores are 3, 2, 4, 4, 4 would receive a median score of 4. However, because these factor scores indicate a minimally critical period and that other people could perform some of tasks, the therapist could recommend a score of 3.

This form does not predetermine service amounts but provides a suggestion based on a typical range for more or less-intensive factors. The IEP team always makes the final determination. Form 4.A has been used for more than 25 years by occupational therapists and physical therapists working in Iowa's schools.

DOCUMENTING OCCUPATIONAL THERAPY INTERVENTIONS

Guidelines for Documentation of Occupational Therapy (AOTA, 2013; see Appendix A) identify common types of therapy documentation reports related to intervention: intervention plans, service contact notes, progress reports, transition plans, and discharge reports. Table 4.4 contains more descriptors about these reports. More detailed information and examples follow.

INTERVENTION PLANS

Although the IEP and the occupation therapy intervention plan both document occupational therapy interventions, there are some important distinctions between the two documents. The *IEP* guides intervention planning and implementation by identifying the student's annual goals for SE and all of the supports and services (including occupational therapy) that will be provided to achieve these goals and to

Table 4.4. COMMON TYPES OF REQUIRED OCCUPATIONAL THERAPY INTERVENTION DOCUMENTATION IN SCHOOLS

FORM NAME	PURPOSE
Intervention plan	Documents intervention goals and strategies used to achieve occupation-based outcomes.
Service contact notes	Documents interactions between the practitioner and student, occupational therapy interventions, student responses, and interventions with others on behalf of the student.
Progress reports	Provides a summary of the intervention process and the student's progress toward identified goals.
Transition plans	Documents the plan for transitioning the student from one setting to another and makes recommendations for services, modifications, and accommodations.
Discharge reports	Provides a summary of the outcomes of occupational therapy services and makes recommendations related to requirements for the future as well as any needed follow-up or referrals.

Source. AOTA (2013).

Table 4.5.   OCCUPATIONAL THERAPY INTERVENTION PLAN USED IN SCHOOLS

COMPONENT	PURPOSE
Client information	Describes important information about the student, including name, birthdate, gender, precautions, and contraindications.
Intervention goals	Identifies measurable and meaningful long- and short-term occupation-based goals that represent the areas of need focused on by occupational therapy.
Intervention approaches and types of interventions	Lists strategies used by the occupational therapy practitioner as defined in the *Framework,* including intervention approaches (e.g., create or promote, establish or restore, maintain, modify, prevent) and types of interventions (e.g., occupations and activities, preparatory methods and tasks, education and training, advocacy, group interventions).
Service delivery mechanisms	Identifies the service providers, location, duration, and frequency of services.
Plan for discharge	Describes the criteria for discontinuation of services or transition to another service setting.
Outcome measures	Identifies the tools that will be used to assess the end result of occupational therapy interventions, including occupational performance, role competence, participation, quality of life, and so on. (See the *Framework* for additional examples of outcomes.)
Professionals responsible and date of plan	Identifies the people monitoring the plan and documents the dates the plan was developed and modified.

Source. AOTA (2013). *Note. Framework = Occupational Therapy Practice Framework: Domain and Process* (AOTA, 2014).

enable the student to participate and make progress in the general education (GE) curriculum. The *occupational therapy intervention plan* directs the actions of the occupational therapy practitioner by outlining the occupation-based goals and occupational therapy interventions.

Although the IEP is developed and reviewed by the IEP team on an annual basis, the occupational therapy intervention plan is a working document that is modified throughout the intervention process (AOTA, 2015). This plan is not part of the IEP. Table 4.5 identifies the suggested components of the occupational therapy intervention plan as described in the *Guidelines for Documentation of Occupational Therapy* (AOTA, 2013).

Form 4.B, "Intervention Plan," provides an intervention plan template. Occupational therapy practitioners often complete this template during or shortly after the IEP meeting. Any services delegated to an occupational therapy assistant should be indicated on this form. As interventions change, this form should be updated.

SERVICE CONTACT NOTES

Service contact notes consist of information about the student and a therapy log that provides a record of occupational therapy interventions. According to the *Guidelines for Documentation*

of Occupational Therapy (AOTA, 2013), the therapy log should include

- Date;
- Type of contact (e.g., phone calls, emails, direct service, meetings with teacher);
- Names or positions of people contacted;
- Client attendance and participation in therapy or reason session was missed;
- Types of interventions implemented and client response;
- Modifications to environment or task;
- Assistive devices created or used;
- Description of education, training, or consultation provided; and
- Current level of client performance.

Occupational therapy services to the student and services on behalf of the student, as well as contacts with others, must be documented. Services to the student include therapeutic use of occupations and activities, preparatory methods, education and training of the student, promoting and supporting student self-advocacy, and group interventions. Services on behalf of the student include education and training of school staff and advocacy efforts to support the student and his or her family.

Service contact notes can be used to manage practitioner workload during interventions. In addition, customized forms can be developed for specific services.

Therapy Log Format

The style of therapy log used may depend on district policies and procedures, types of interventions, and practitioner preferences. Table 4.6 provides descriptions of some common therapy log formats that can be used to record both hands-on services and services on behalf of the student. Here, we discuss three types of therapy logs: (1) written or electronic service record that combines an attendance log with a therapy log, (2) column-style service log, and (3) flow sheet.

Written or electronic service record with attendance log

Form 4.C, "Service Record," provides a written or electronic record of student demographics and IEP data. The attendance log at the bottom of the first page allows the practitioner to see at a quick glance what contacts have been made each month (e.g., intervention, evaluation, meetings, telephone, electronic contact). The next page (which can be used as ongoing pages as needed) allows practitioners to document the data, time (time in and out can be recorded, if needed for agency records), a record of the intervention, meeting information, contacts, and so on.

Column-style service log

Form 4.D, "Column Notes," provides an example of column-style notes, another method of documenting interventions and the ongoing plan. This form allows practitioners to record interventions and notes manually or electronically. These student forms should be kept confidential and easily accessible to the occupational therapy practitioners.

Flow sheet

Form 4.E, "Flow Sheet," provides an example of a flow sheet. This method of recording therapy activities helps streamline the documentation process when the therapy session follows a consistent format from one session to the next. The flow of the session (or lesson plan) is recorded in the column on the left, and the student's responses are recorded in the date columns to the right. This form is an example of a flow sheet used for a weekly social skills group that began with an opening activity (review from the previous week), then a movement-based warm-up activity, followed by the lesson (introduction of the topic, demonstration, and role playing), a self-calming exercise, and a closing activity.

A flow sheet might also be useful for a preschool motor group in which the students rotate through the same four stations each week (e.g., balance, ball skills, scooter boards, locomotor skills) or a monthly consultation meeting in which the same general topics are discussed (e.g., updates on student performance, current concerns, program modifications, plan for follow-up).

Managing Workload During Intervention

To manage your workload during intervention, recording the students' demographic information in a caseload list is beneficial (see Form 4.F, "Caseload List"). The caseload list can also be used to provide data for a mail-merge document.

Form 4.G, "Annual Review Sheet," can be used as a quick guide for tracking upcoming annual reviews for students. For instance, add the dates as you learn of a student's review

Table 4.6. COMMON THERAPY LOG FORMATS IN SCHOOLS

FORMAT	DESCRIPTION	COMMENTS
Attendance log	Contains the days of the school year and spaces to record minutes, types of contacts, absences, and reason for absences.	• Summarizes attendance for the year on 1 page. • Provides limited information; typically used in combination with another form.
SOAP notes	Contains *subjective* information, *objective* observations, *assessment* or analysis of subjective and objective information, and *plans* for continued therapy interventions.	• Provides detailed information. • Can be difficult to find specific performance data for data analysis and progress reporting.
Column notes	Information is separated into 3 or more columns (e.g., date, activity/intervention, response, plan).	• Columns allow quick review to find performance data, when staff were trained on a specific procedure, ideas for next therapy session, and so on.
Flow sheet	Therapy notes are recorded in a table with the therapy activities completed in a typical session listed in the column on the left; dated columns to the right provide space for recording client response to each therapy activity during the session.	• Useful when the therapy session or consultation meeting follows the same general format from session to session. • Quick to fill out but may provide limited qualitative information.

Table 4.7.   DOCUMENTATION FORMS FOR SERVICES ON BEHALF OF THE STUDENT

FORM	DESCRIPTION	EXAMPLES OF USE
Procedural checklist	Includes a list of procedures or steps that need to be followed to carry out a particular task; may also include a place for trainee to initial or sign to acknowledge receipt of training.	OTA completes the form while training staff on how to safely position a student with multiple complex health needs.
Equipment use guidelines	Explains how the equipment is used and any precautions or contraindications for use of the equipment; may also include a place for trainee to initial or sign to acknowledge receipt of training.	OT completes the form while providing training regarding how and when to use an adaptive keyboard in the classroom.
Consultation report form	Documents reason for consultation, areas of concern, therapist observations, suggestions or recommendations, and follow-up needed.	OT completes the form to document job site consultation and suggestions for activity modifications for a student in a school-to-work transition program.
Fidelity rating scale (see Chapter 2, "Data Collection," for examples)	Records the extent to which interventions are implemented by another person.	The form is provided to the teacher to record how well he or she is able to implement a student's feeding program.
Parent communication form	Documents contacts between practitioner and family.	The form is provided to the parent to share information about the student or program.

Note. OT = occupational therapist; OTA = occupational therapy assistant.

(e.g., under "September," add 15–Liam A., November 10–Stella C.). Then you can organize your workload in order to have reevaluations and other tasks completed by those dates.

Customized Forms

Some services on behalf of the student, such as training in specific procedures, provision of specialized equipment, or formal consultations, may be documented more effectively using customized forms that can then be shared with the student receiving the intervention. Table 4.7 provides descriptions of some supplemental forms that can be used to document services on behalf of the student and provide written documentation to the person receiving the services.

Form 4.H, "Consultation Report Form," can be used when consulting with a teacher for a student on an IEP. The form documents occupational therapy services and provides written feedback to the teacher. If follow-up observations or interventions are provided, they can be documented on the second page of the form.

Form 4.I, "Eating/Feeding Plan," illustrates a feeding plan for a student who has significant feeding issues. This is a type of procedural checklist and can be used by anyone who feeds a student to increase safety.

Form 4.J, "Documentation of School Food Modifications," is a procedural checklist used to ensure a student's school food (e.g., breakfast, lunch, snack) is properly modified by the cafeteria. Some districts have a form and policy about such modifications (e.g., require a physician's signature). This form may be included as part of the student's 504 Plan or IEP.

PROGRESS REPORTS

In schools, occupational therapy practitioners provide progress reports in accordance with IDEA requirements that periodic reports on progress toward IEP goals are provided to parents at the same time report cards are issued (§1414[d][1][A][IV]). Progress reports typically are provided every quarter or trimester. The format for progress reports is often determined by the school district and may be embedded within the IEP software used by the local education agency. Sometimes a graph can be used to visually convey the progress to parents (see Form 4.K, "Sample Quarterly Progress Note to Parent" about Daisy).

Daisy is an 8-year-old student who attends an elementary school and receives self-contained programming with integration into GE. Eating and chewing skills are very delayed because of Daisy's cerebral palsy, and she often coughs and gags on food, which causes it to fly out of her mouth as well as increase her risk of aspiration. Her parents were resistant to changing her diet of mashed foods to a blended diet, but they agreed after consulting with medical staff. The parents wanted to continue feeding Daisy orally even though a gastrostomy tube would be easier for nutritional intake.

The school dietitian blends Daisy's food separately. The teacher or associate noticed that certain blended foods and milk were still difficult for Daisy and were likely to cause her to choke or gag. Her parents agreed to substitutes for some of the foods (e.g., blended hamburger, tacos) but requested milk not be removed. After the first month, when her program was reviewed, it was clear that the progress was not proceeding as fast as needed for her to meet her goal (e.g., comparing the

Table 4.8. COMPARISON OF TRANSITION PLAN CONTENT

SUGGESTED TRANSITION PLAN CONTENT (AOTA, 2013)	IDEA REQUIREMENTS FOR TRANSITION PLANS (34 CFR §300.320[B])

• Client information
• Current status of the client
• Plan for transition, including
  ○ Current setting and transition setting
  ○ Reason for transition
  ○ Time frame of the transition
  ○ Activities to be completed to support the transition
• Recommendations (e.g., accommodations, modifications, assistive technology)
	• Measurable postsecondary goals related to
	  ○ Training
	  ○ Education
	  ○ Employment
	  ○ Independent living skills (when appropriate)
	• Transition services (including courses of study) needed to help the student achieve goals

data to solid black goal line in Form 4.K). Daisy's parents agreed to try removal of the milk for a month to see how Daisy performed. Sending home the graph allowed the family to see her actual performance during lunch (measured daily, but only Wednesday data are graphed on Form 4.K).

According to AOTA (2013), progress reports provide a summary of the intervention process and documentation of the client's progress toward goal achievement. Suggested content of the progress report includes

- Client information (e.g., name, birthdate, gender, diagnosis)
- Summary of occupational therapy services, including
  - Frequency of services and how long services have been provided
  - Measurable progress or lack of progress
  - Modifications to task or environment
  - Adaptive equipment
  - Relevant client updates
  - Client response to occupational therapy interventions
  - Client or caregiver training.
- Current progress on goals and occupational performance
- Plan or recommendations.

Some occupational therapy practitioners complete an annual progress report that includes a summary of the student's occupational therapy services and suggestions in addition to progress on goals. This annual report could be completed at the time of the student's annual review so that the data may be used in planning for the next IEP. A sample format for an annual progress report is included in Form 4.L, "Annual Progress or Discharge Report," which typically is a one-page report summarizing the student's background, performance, services provided, and plans for ongoing occupational therapy services.

TRANSITION PLANS

Under IDEA, transition plans are a mandated part of the IEP for students turning 16 (or younger in some states; 34 CFR

§300.320[b]). They provide a description of the supports, services, and specially designed instruction needed to prepare the student for life after graduation. These transition plans differ from the description of transition plans provided by AOTA (2013), which focuses on how the client will transition from one service setting to another. Occupational therapy practitioners who support school-based transition programs may complete a discharge summary and contribute to the summary of performance required under IDEA for students who are no longer eligible for services because of age or graduation (see the "Discharge Reports" section for additional information). Table 4.8 compares the content of the transition plan suggested in the *Guidelines for Documentation of Occupational Therapy* (AOTA, 2013) with the transition plan requirements of IDEA.

DISCHARGE REPORTS

Discontinuing occupational therapy may be suggested when any one of the following criteria are met:

- Goal is no longer educationally relevant.
- Goal was met and no additional goals that require occupational therapy intervention are appropriate.
- Continued occupational therapy intervention is unlikely to result in benefit to the student.
- Skills and expertise of the occupational therapy practitioner are no longer needed to meet the student's educational needs (e.g., needs can be met through other team resources).
- Therapy is contraindicated because of medical or health, psychological, or physical status.
- Parents decline ongoing goals in that area.

An example of a goal no longer being educationally relevant occurs when a student has struggled with cutting and coloring but, as he enters a higher grade level, those skills are no longer relevant because they occur seldom in the program. The IEP goal is no longer educationally relevant. The fourth

Table 4.9. COMPARISON OF DISCHARGE REPORT AND SUMMARY OF PERFORMANCE

SUGGESTED DISCHARGE REPORT CONTENT (AOTA, 2013)	IDEA SUMMARY OF PERFORMANCE REQUIREMENTS (34 CFR §300.305[E])

• Client information
• Summary of the intervention process
  ○ Dates of initial and final service
  ○ Frequency of services and number of sessions
  ○ Summary of therapy interventions
  ○ Summary of progress toward goals
  ○ Outcomes of occupational therapy (change in status of occupational engagement, client's and family's perception of the effectiveness of occupational therapy services)
• Recommendations related to the future needs of the client as well as a plan for follow-up or referrals to other services if needed
	• Summary of the child's academic achievement and functional performance
	• Recommendations for how to help the child meet his or her postsecondary goals

bullet reflects the instance of an occupational therapist who has provided the teacher with pertinent knowledge and skills and the teacher is able to carry out the program without ongoing support from an occupational therapist. For example, a student with severe intellectual impairment may have struggled learning to drink from a cup and received occupational therapy services to meet this IEP goal. A year later, at the annual IEP review, the student has made progress but has not mastered the skill. The teacher and classroom paraprofessional have been implementing the cup-drinking program developed by the occupational therapist. There is no additional need for the occupational therapist to be involved; however, the student goal continues to be a priority and will remain on the IEP.

In cases such as the ones just listed, a discharge report may be completed. The *discharge report* provides a summary of how the client's occupational performance has changed from the initial evaluation to time of discharge and offers recommendations as appropriate (AOTA, 2013). Under IDEA, a reevaluation is required before a change in eligibility status is made, unless the student graduates with a regular diploma or the student's age exceeds the age of eligibility for a free appropriate public education. For these students, the district must provide a summary of performance (34 CFR §300.305[e]). Table 4.9 compares the content of the discharge report suggested in the *Guidelines for Documentation of Occupational Therapy* (AOTA, 2013) with the content of the summary of performance required by IDEA.

A discharge summary report is similar to the annual progress report (see Form 4.L), but instead of describing plans for ongoing occupational therapy services, the discharge summary report provides a rationale for terminating services and offers suggestions or recommendations to support ongoing student success. Form 4.M, "Sample Annual Progress or Discharge Report," provides a description of how Form 4.L is used. In some cases, it may also be appropriate to provide guidance regarding when to reconsider the need for occupational therapy. Sometimes the decision to discontinue occupational therapy services coincides with the student's 3-year reevaluation. In that case, this

information would be included within the reevaluation report (see Chapter 3, "Tiered Support: Screening and Evaluation").

SUMMARY

Documentation of occupational therapy intervention planning, implementation, review, and discharge is an essential part of the occupational therapy process that provides a legal record of what was done. Intervention plans and consistent documentation of occupational therapy interventions guide therapy decision making, and progress reports, annual reports, and discharge summaries help communicate to others the impact of occupational therapy services on student progress.

REFERENCES

American Occupational Therapy Association. (2013). Guidelines for documentation of occupational therapy. *American Journal of Occupational Therapy, 67*(Suppl.), S32–S38. https://doi.org/10.5014/ajot.2013.67S32

American Occupational Therapy Association. (2014). Occupational therapy practice framework: Domain and process (3rd ed.). *American Journal of Occupational Therapy, 68*(Suppl. 1), S1–S48. https://doi.org/10.5014/ajot.2014.682006

American Occupational Therapy Association. (2015). Standards of practice for occupational *therapy. American Journal of Occupational Therapy, 69*(Suppl. 3), 1–6. https://doi.org/10.5014/ajot.2015.696S06

Frolek Clark, G. (2013). Best practices in school occupational therapy documentation. In G. Frolek Clark & B. Chandler (Eds.), *Best practices for occupational therapy in schools* (pp. 107–119). Bethesda, MD: AOTA Press.

Individuals with Disabilities Education Improvement Act of 2004, Pub L. 108–446, 20 U.S.C. §1400-1482.

FORM 4.A. RANGE OF SERVICE GUIDELINES

Student: _____   Birthdate: _____

Purpose: These guidelines are used for making recommendations regarding the frequency and duration of services. The Range of Service Suggested section should be reviewed at least annually.

Directions: Circle or highlight one statement in each row that best describes the student's current status.

Decision: Must be a whole number based on **median score** (NOT the average). Use your professional judgment.

Example: If the row scores are 2, 3, 3, 2, then student score is 2; if the row scores are 3,4,4,2,1, then student score is 3.

Factors	1	2	3	4
Potential to benefit with therapeutic intervention	Student demonstrates minimal potential for change.	Student appears to have potential for change but at a slower rate.	Student appears to have a significant potential for change.	Student appears to have a high potential to improve skills.
Critical period of skill acquisition or regression related to development or disability	Not a critical period.	Minimally critical period.	Critical period.	Extremely critical period.
Amount of program that can be performed by others in addition to therapist intervention	Program can be carried out safely by others with periodic intervention by therapist.	Many activities from the program can be safely performed by others in addition to intervention by therapist.	Some activities from the program can be safely performed by others in addition to intervention by therapist.	A few activities can be safely performed by others, but most of the program requires the expertise of the therapist.
Amount of training provided by therapist to others carrying out the program	Teacher, staff, and/or parents highly trained to meet student's needs. No additional training needed.	Teacher, staff, and/or parents trained but some follow-up needed.	Teacher, staff, and/or parents could be trained to carry out some activities.	Teacher, staff, and/or parents could carry out some activities with extensive training.
Amount problem interferes with education setting	Environment is accommodating, and difficulties are minimal.	Environment is accommodating, and difficulties are moderately interfering.	Environment is accommodating, but difficulties are significant.	Environment is not accommodating, or environment is accommodating, but problems are severe.
Range of Service Suggested	1	2	3	4
OT Services				
PT Services				

Note. OT = occupational therapy; PT = physical therapy. The range of service minutes for each number on the scale is determined by the occupational therapy departments based on the range of services provided within the district. Reprinted with permission from Gloria Frolek Clark. Developed before 1990 with collaboration from Kathy David, PT, when they were consultants for the Iowa Department of Education, and with feedback from the State OT & PT Lead Group.

FORM 4.B. INTERVENTION PLAN

Occupational Therapy Intervention Plan

Client information			
Name:		Date of birth:	School and grade:
District:	Parents:	Phone:	

Diagnosis or conditions:

Precautions:

Intervention goals—Check and describe areas of occupations to be addressed
☐ ADLs   ☐ IADLs   ☐ Education   ☐ Leisure   ☐ Play   ☐ Rest and sleep   ☐ Social participation   ☐ Work

Intervention approaches—Check and describe
☐ Create/promote   ☐ Establish/Restore   ☐ Maintain   ☐ Modify   ☐ Prevent

Types of interventions—Check and describe
☐ Occupations and activities   ☐ Preparatory methods and tasks   ☐ Education and training   ☐ Advocacy   ☐ Group

Service delivery mechanisms	
Frequency:	Duration:
Location of services:	Provider(s):

Discharge plan (criteria for discharge)

Outcome measures (check)
☐ Occupational performance   ☐ Prevention   ☐ Health and wellness   ☐ Quality of life
☐ Participation   ☐ Role competence   ☐ Well-being   ☐ Occupational justice

Developed by:

Date developed: **Date revised:**

Note. ADLs = activities of daily living; IADLs = instrumental activities of daily living.

FORM 4.C. SERVICE RECORD

Occupational Therapy
Service Record

SERVICE RECORD BEGINNING _____ ENDING _____

Student: _____ Date of Birth: _____ Age: _____

Parents: _____ Phone: _____

Address: _____ Email: _____

School District: _____ Building: _____

Teacher(s): _____ Grade: _____ FBA/BIP Yes ☐ No ☐

Case Manager: _____ Contact: _____

OT Frequency and Duration on IEP: _____

Review Dates: Annual review: _____ 3-year review: _____

Medical Conditions or Precautions: _____

LOG OF CONTACT DATES

Directions: List the month this log was started. List the date, and use the key to indicate the service or contact. Provide documentation of these events on the following sheets.

Month   Month

Service key: C = cancellation; E = evaluations; EC = electronic contact; I = interventions; M = meeting/conference; T = telephone.

Note. BIP = behavior intervention plan; FBA = functional behavior assessment; IEP = individualized education program; OT = occupational therapy.

Occupational Therapy
Service Record (Electronic Version)

SERVICE RECORD BEGINNING _____   **ENDING** _____

Student: _____   Date of Birth: _____   Age: _____

Directions: Enter the data as well as the time for services.

Date:	Time:
Notes:	
Electronic signature:	

Date:	Time:
Notes:	
Electronic signature:	

Date:	Time:
Notes:	
Electronic signature:	

Date:	Time:
Notes:	
Electronic signature:	

FORM 4.D. COLUMN NOTES

Occupational Therapy Notes

Student: **IEP Date:**   **Therapist:**

Date	Interventions	Notes	Plan
	☐ Occupations/Activities ☐ Preparatory Methods/Tasks ☐ Education/Training ☐ Groups Describe:		
	☐ Occupations/Activities ☐ Preparatory Methods/Tasks ☐ Education/Training ☐ Groups Describe:		
	☐ Occupations/Activities ☐ Preparatory Methods/Tasks ☐ Education/Training ☐ Groups Describe:		
	☐ Occupations/Activities ☐ Preparatory Methods/Tasks ☐ Education/Training ☐ Groups Describe:		

Note. IEP = individualized education program.

FORM 4.E. FLOW SHEET

Therapy Group Flow Sheet

Student Name: _____   IEP Date: _____   Therapist: _____

Goals: _____

Date				
Opening				
Warm-ups				
Lesson or activity				
Calming				
Closing				

FORM 4.F. CASELOAD LIST

Therapist Name: _____

School Year: _____

Caseload List

Last Name	First Name	Date of Birth	Age	Grade	Disability Category	IEP Due Date	Evaluation Due Date	OT Minutes of Service	Teacher Name	School

Disability Categories:

DD – Developmental Disability	ASD – Autism	DB – Deaf-Blindness	D – Deafness
MD – Multiple Disabilities	ED – Emotional Disturbance	HI – Hearing Impairment	ID – Intellectual Disability
SLI – Speech/Language Impairment	OI – Orthopedic Impairment	OHI – Other Health Impairments	SLD – Specific Learning Disability
	TBI – Traumatic Brain Injury	VI – Visual Impairment	

Note. IEP = individualized education program; OT = occupational therapy.

FORM 4.G. ANNUAL REVIEW SHEET

Annual Review Schedule

Staff Member: _____   School Year: _____

Directions: According to the student's IEP annual review, place the date and student's name (or initials) under the appropriate month.

August	September	October	November	December	January

February	March	April	May	June	July

Note. IEP = individualized education program.

FORM 4.H. CONSULTATION REPORT FORM

Occupational Therapy
Consultation Report Form

Student Name: _____ Date of Birth: _____

School: _____ Age: _____ Grade: _____

Therapist: _____ Observation Date(s): _____

Concerns/background:

Observation summary:

Suggestions:

Follow-up plan:

Signed: _____ Date: _____

Occupational Therapy
Consultation Report Form
- Page 2 -

Follow-up Date: _____

Observations/Discussion:

Suggestions/Follow-Up:

Signed: _____ Date: _____

Follow-up date: _____

Observations/Discussion:

Suggestions/Follow-Up:

Signed: _____ Date: _____

Follow-up date: _____

Observations/Discussion:

Suggestions/Follow-Up:

Signed: _____ Date: _____

FORM 4.I. EATING/FEEDING PLAN

Eating/Feeding Plan

Student's Name: _____   Birthdate: _____

Date Developed: _____   Reviewed: _____

Parent and Teacher Participation in Plan: _____

Topic	Instructions
Prior to feeding	
Precautions known	
Positioning and equipment	
Liquid textures	☐ Nectar (e.g., strained fruit juice) ☐ Thickened liquids
Food textures	☐ Pureed foods (no lumps, applesauce) ☐ Thickened pureed (small lumps with liquid, yogurt) ☐ Blended table foods (minimal liquid added) ☐ Mashed foods (mashed with fork, some lumps, minimal liquid) ☐ Ground foods (no liquids added, hamburger) ☐ Chopped foods (cut to approximately ¼ in.)
Eating procedure	
Drinking procedure	
OT name and contact information	

Note. OT = occupational therapist.

FORM 4.J. DOCUMENTATION OF SCHOOL FOOD MODIFICATIONS

School Food Modification Plan

Student: _____   Birthdate: _____

School: _____   Date: _____

Known medical conditions:

Reason for modifications:

A. Modifications needed (check all that apply):

☐ Substitute menu items (i.e., allergy, substitution for foods that don't puree well) _____

☐ Texture modifications (check ones that apply):

Liquids
_____   Nectar: liquids that have some "texture" (e.g., tomato juice, strained fruit/juice)
_____   Thick liquids: liquids that have been thickened

Foods
_____   Pureed foods: semi-solid (no lumps), high water content (e.g., applesauce, baby food)
_____   Thickened pureed foods: semi-solid (small lumps).
_____   Blenderized table foods with minimal liquid added (e.g., mashed potato, yogurt, pudding)
_____   Ground foods: Table foods in grinder/blender, NO liquids added (e.g., hamburger)
_____   Chopped foods: Table foods cut to approximately 1/4 of an inch

☐ Recipe modifications (i.e., low fat, low sugar, high fiber) _____

☐ Other modifications (i.e., temperature, portion size, nutrient enhancers) _____

B. Certification from physician:

I certify that the above food modification is necessary for this student because of medical or special dietary needs.

Physician's Signature: _____   Date: _____

Physician: _____   Phone: _____

FORM 4.K. SAMPLE QUARTERLY PROGRESS NOTE TO PARENT

Lincoln School District
School Year: 2016–2017

Progress Report: Quarter 1st _X_ 2nd ____ 3rd ____ 4th ____

Student's Name: Daisy   Birthdate: 11-1-06

GOAL: During the school lunch, when blended foods and thickened liquids are presented, Daisy will eat at least 50% of the lunch, without gagging or choking more than twice per meal.

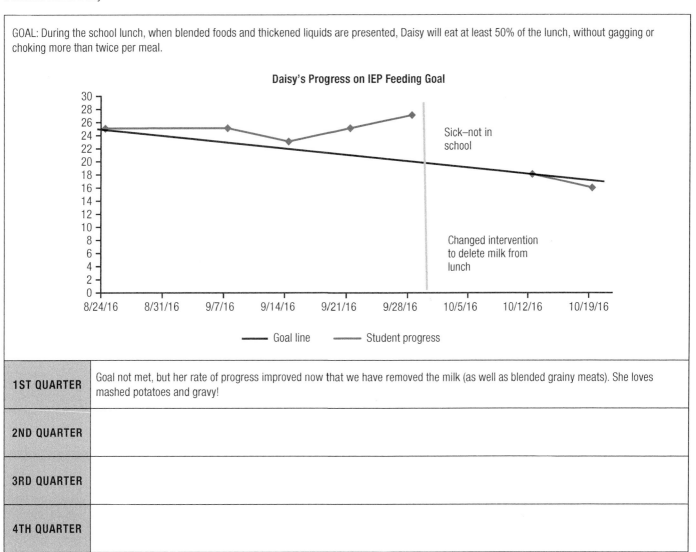

Daisy's Progress on IEP Feeding Goal

1ST QUARTER	Goal not met, but her rate of progress improved now that we have removed the milk (as well as blended grainy meats). She loves mashed potatoes and gravy!
2ND QUARTER	
3RD QUARTER	
4TH QUARTER	

FORM 4.L. ANNUAL PROGRESS OR DISCHARGE REPORT

Occupational Therapy
(Annual Progress Report or Discharge Summary)

Student: _____ Date of Birth: _____ Grade: _____

Attending District: _____ Attending Building: _____

Report Written By: _____ Date: _____

Background information: Can include information about the initial referral and educational or health information that is significant.

[ ]

Summary of service provided: Can summarize the area of focus, frequency of occupational therapy services, types of intervention and approaches used, participation of parents and teacher, and so on.

[ ]

Current status: Can share information about the student's current performance, new concerns, and equipment or materials needed.

[ ]

Plan or recommendations: Can share ongoing plans or suggestions. If services are ongoing, list the focus of services, suggested training, future transitions, and so on. If services are not ongoing, discuss exit planning.

[ ]

FORM 4.M. SAMPLE ANNUAL PROGRESS OR DISCHARGE REPORT

Occupational Therapy
Progress Note and Suggested Discharge

Name: <u>Ethan P.</u>   Date of Birth: _____   Date: _____

Attending District: _____   Attending Building: <u>Elementary</u>_____

Report Written By: _____

Background Information

Ethan received occupational therapy services during early intervention and in preschool. Currently, he attends full-day kindergarten and receives special education and related services (e.g., resource teacher and an occupational therapist) in his general education (GE) classroom. Ethan has a medical diagnosis of cerebral palsy (had a shunt placed at age 7 months). He is able to use his nondominant (right) hand to spontaneously hold/stabilize objects while manipulating them with his left, dominant hand. There is some tightness in his left forearm; however, he practices turning his palm up during the day (e.g., lunch card placed on palm, receives "high five" from peers).

Summary of Services Provided

This year our focus has been on Ethan's participation in the GE classroom with emphasis on completing his fine motor and written language tasks. He has received weekly services for 30 minutes for the first 2 months of the school year and then the frequency was changed to 30 minutes every 2 weeks due to improved performance and ability of teachers to incorporate strategies into the daily program, which provided him with daily practice. His parents are very committed to Ethan's progress and communication between home and school occurs at least weekly. He has been very cooperative during intervention sessions, and his parents and teachers have implemented suggestions and strategies from the occupational therapist.

Current Performance

Goal: By 2/14/17, during fine motor and written language activities in his classroom, Ethan will complete the 90% of the activities independently for 3 consecutive days.

At this time, Ethan has managed to perform 80% of these skills independently. During classroom activities, he can cut out shapes, write his name on papers, and copy diagonal lines and basic shapes. The "X" is sometimes 1 diagonal and 1 vertical line, but he does notice it isn't correct and tries to fix this. Three weeks ago, he wrote 18 of the capital letters from a model. Two weeks ago, this occupational therapist reviewed written classroom samples from Ethan and 6 classroom peers (classroom writing sample). All had used the same sheets and copied the capital letters from a model. Median score across these peers is 23/26 (88.5%). Ethan performed 15/26 (median score is 15; 57.7%).

Peer 1—24/26; Peer 2—26/26; Peer 3—26/26; Peer 4—19/26; Peer 5—20/26; Peer 6—22/26.

Ethan continues to demonstrate a delay in copying his alphabet due to distractibility and not completing classroom work. The resource room teacher will assist in strategies for work completion. His performance fluctuates depending upon his motivation, but he has demonstrated the skills to complete this work.

Plans or Recommendations

Ethan has made significant gains but continues to need instruction in the area of written language. His resource room teacher is knowledgeable in this area and will work on advanced literacy skills. At this time, discontinuation of occupational therapy services is suggested.

5

Outcomes and Program Evaluation

P rogram evaluation may be completed at the individual level (i.e., did occupational therapy services make a difference for this student?), population level (i.e., are occupational therapy services effective for students in this school district? Did occupational therapy services make a difference for students across this agency?), and department level (i.e., are all therapists completing intervention plans for students receiving services? Are all of the necessary forms being completed in the occupational therapist's working file for each student?). To evaluate these programs and make decisions, data collection is important. Using forms that make data collection easy as well as reliable and valid is critical.

STUDENT OUTCOMES

"*Outcomes* of occupational therapy services provided for school-aged children are most often measured by achievement of targeted [individualized education program] goals for individual students" (Argabrite Grove, 2013, p. 124). Although occupational therapists are involved in both general education (GE) and other areas, data can be gathered to answer one question: "Are occupational therapy services effective for students in this school district?" Completing a form, such as Form 5.A, "Districtwide Program Evaluation of Students Receiving Occupational Therapy on an IEP," during a school year can provide data for the analysis of a program's strengths and needs. Decisions based on these data can be made for the following year.

Table 5.1.   EXAMPLE OF FORM 5.A COMPLETED FOR TWO STUDENTS

ENTER MONTH OF ANNUAL REVIEW (E.G., 01, 02)	ENTER STUDENT INITIALS (FIRST INITIAL, LAST INITIAL)	ENTER GRADE	ENTER IEP GOAL CODE (ONE CODE PER LINE)	ENTER GOAL STATUS CODE	ENTER OTHERS ON THIS GOAL
09	TG	PS	1	M	2
	Same		8	NM	2
09	BB	G3	6	M	3

Note. IEP = individualized education program.

For example, after each student's annual individualized education program meeting, the status of the goals is recorded on the form (see Table 5.1). If a student met his or her goal, an "M" would be placed in the relevant box. When a student had two goals that occupational therapist has been addressing (e.g., 1–dressing; 8–functional motor skills), then two lines are used. Writing "Same" on the second line of the form prevents that student from being counted twice (e.g., Table 5.1 lists information for 2 students and 3 goals).

Data from Form 5.A can then be summarized, analyzed, and reported as shown in Exhibit 5.1. Although this sample report page does not show the results of each of the categories, we recommend that a completed report share all of these data. Distributing an annual report to stakeholders, to provide them with information about the effectiveness of occupational therapy services, is also recommended.

DOCUMENTATION OUTCOMES

To evaluate occupational therapy documentation in the schools, a question may be posed, such as, "Are all of the necessary forms being completed in the occupational therapist's working file for each student?" Form 5.B, "Program Evaluation of Occupational Therapy Documentation," was designed to help answer that question. The various forms listed on Form 5.B are only suggestions and will be determined by your agency's policies.

Program evaluation can be used to develop consistent practices for occupational therapy practitioners within a school district and to create common forms and documentation (McKinley-Vargas & Thomas, 2008). To begin program evaluation, generate and then prioritize your questions. Determine which ones you want to address this year. Then develop data collection sheets and get started. You may want to collect data for several years

to determine changes (e.g., student grades, number of students referred), but other data could be collected every 2 years, which allows different information to be collected on the alternating years. For example, the first-year's data collection would focus on GE and special education (SE) students; however, the second-year's data collection would focus on SE students and occupational therapy department documentation.

STAFF TIME STUDY

Another program evaluation tool is a *time study* in which data are collected regarding how much time occupational therapy practitioners spend doing their assigned tasks, including providing services to support eligible students under the Individuals with Disabilities Education Improvement Act of 2004 (P. L. 108–446; both services to the child and those on behalf of the child) and other duties, such as conducting evaluations, attending team meetings, and providing early intervening services. Time study data can be used to determine the capacity for occupational therapy services in the school district and to advocate for additional therapy staff (Jackson, 2013; Polichino & Jackson, 2014).

To complete a time study, occupational therapy practitioners identify all of their assigned tasks, select a time increment (e.g., 15 minutes) and determine a data collection schedule (e.g., 2 weeks in October, February, and May). Each practitioner in the district then records his or her activities following the schedule, and the resulting data are analyzed. Form 5.C, "Example Time Study Data Form," provides an example of a time study data collection form. An excellent example of a spreadsheet data form developed by Jodie Williams, OTR/L, MHA, and Susan Cecere, PT, MHS, was shared on the OTConnections online Early Intervention and Schools Special Interest Section forum (Williams, 2012). OTConnections, a professional

Exhibit 5.1.   SAMPLE REPORT OF EFFECTIVENESS

Effectiveness of Occupational Therapy: Meeting Students' IEP Goals
School Year 2016–17

Number of Students	During the School Year 2016–17, occupational therapists and occupational therapy assistants in Happy Student School District served 210 students in SE students. This is an increase of 15% in the past years.
Goal Outcomes	A total of 210 students received occupational therapy services on their IEP. At their annual IEP meeting, the status of their goal was reviewed with team members. The majority of goals were met (M), not met but significantly improved (NM), or advanced goals were written (A). Some students made limited progress (LP), and others were not in the system due to moving or graduating (X).

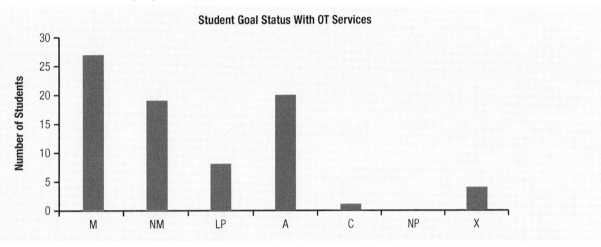

Note. This is a sample only; factual data were not used. C = continue as written; IEP = individualized education program; NP = goal area not a priority at this time; OT = occupational therapy; SE = special education.

networking resource available through the American Occupational Therapy Association (AOTA) offers public forums, AOTA and community blogs, and member forums. (*Note.* At the time of press, AOTA members can access the time study data collection form by logging on to OTConnections, typing "Buzzing About Workload vs. Caseload" into the search field, and selecting the thread titled "Buzzing About Workload vs. Caseload" under "Forums." The spreadsheet, titled "Time Study daily.xls," is attached to the second post in the thread.)

SUMMARY

There are many reasons to conduct a program evaluation (e.g., to identify how occupational therapy practitioners are using their time, to determine effectiveness of meeting student outcomes, to determine whether department paperwork is complete, to identify strengths and needs within the department). Designing a document to gather these data is essential. Sharing the results of the program evaluation allows others (e.g., administrators, colleagues) to understand more about occupational therapy services.

REFERENCES

Argabrite Grove, R. (2013). Best practices in school occupational therapy program evaluation. In G. Frolek Clark & B. Chandler (Eds.), *Best practices for occupational therapy in schools* (pp. 121–129). Bethesda, MD: AOTA Press.

Individuals with Disabilities Education Improvement Act of 2004, Pub L. 108–446, 20 U.S.C. § 1400–1482.

Jackson, L. (2013). Best practices in determining school workloads. In G. Frolek Clark & B. Chandler (Eds.), *Best practices for occupational therapy in schools* (pp. 131–139). Bethesda, MD: AOTA Press.

McKinley-Vargas, J., & Thomas, K. (2008, June 30). A framework for change. *OT Practice, 13*(11), 10–15.

Polichino, J., & Jackson, L. (2014). *Transforming caseload to workload in school-based occupational therapy services.* Retrieved from http://www.aota.org/~/media/Corporate/Files/Secure/Practice/Children/Workload-fact.pdf

Williams, J. (2012, May 7). Buzzing about workload vs caseload [Online forum comment]. *Early Intervention and School Special Interest Section Forum, OT Connections.* Retrieved from https://otconnections.aota.org/sis_forums/f/17/t/14350.aspx

FORM 5.A. DISTRICTWIDE PROGRAM EVALUATION OF STUDENTS RECEIVING OCCUPATIONAL THERAPY ON AN IEP

Therapist Name: _____   School Year: _____

Directions: After the student's annual review during current school year, complete the information on students receiving service on an IEP. Enter data for each student's IEP goal that OT addresses using 1 line per IEP goal code. Only use codes from box below.

Column	Descriptions/Codes
Month of review	Enter the month that the annual review is due (date on IEP or agency form).
Student initials	Enter student's initials (first initial then last initial).
Grade	Enter code: PS = preschool; K = kindergarten; G1 = Grade 1; G2 = Grade 2, and so on.
IEP goal code	Enter code: *Self-care:* 1 = dressing; 2 = feeding or eating; 3 = hygiene, grooming, or toileting. *Education:* 4 = access and participation; 5 = attention; 6 = literacy–writing; 7 = literacy–reading; 8 = fine motor skills; 9 = large motor skills; 10 = organization; 11 = prevocation; 12 = play or leisure; 13 = social participation. *Other:* 14 = (describe in 1–3 words) _____.
Goal status code	Enter code: M = met goal; NM = not met but improved significantly; LP = limited progress; A = more advanced work in goal area; C = continue as written; NP = goal area not a priority at this time; X = if student gone (e.g., moved, graduated, died).
Others on this goal	Enter code: 1 = OT only person working on this goal; 2 = OT plus teacher (e.g., GE teacher, SE teacher, PS teacher); 3 = OT plus teacher and parent; 4 = OT and parent; 5 = OT and PT or SLP only; 6 = multiple team members.

Enter Month of Annual Review (e.g., 01, 02)	Enter Student Initials	Enter Grade	Enter IEP Goal Code (1 Code Per Line)	Enter Goal Status Code	Enter Others on This Goal

Note. GE = general education; IEP = individualized education program; PS = preschool; PT = physical therapist; OT = occupational therapist; SE = special education; SLP = speech–language pathologist.

FORM 5.B. PROGRAM EVALUATION OF OCCUPATIONAL THERAPY DOCUMENTATION

Therapist Name: _____   **School Year:** _____

Directions: Check boxes if the forms are present and appropriately completed for each student in the occupational therapy working file.

Enter Student Initials (first initial, last initial)	Current OT Evaluation Report	OT Intervention Plan	Service Contact Notes	Progress Reports	Data Sheet	Copies of Current Goal Pages That Include OT Service

Note. OT = occupational therapy.

FORM 5.C. EXAMPLE TIME STUDY DATA FORM

Therapist Code: _____   Date: _____

Time	Monday	Tuesday	Wednesday	Thursday	Friday
8:00 A.M.					
8:15					
8:30					
8:45					
9:00					
9:15					
9:30					
9:45					
10:00					
10:15					
10:30					
10:45					
11:00					
11:15					
11:30					
11:45					
12:00 P.M.					
12:15					
12:30					
12:45					
1:00					
1:15					
1:30					
1:45					
2:00					
2:15					
2:30					
2:45					
3:00					
3:15					
3:30					
3:45					
4:00					
4:15					

Directions: Enter the appropriate code for each 15-minute increment.

D = direct services	I = indirect services	EIS = early intervening services
Ev = evaluation	M = team meeting	PD = professional development
T = travel time	S = supervision/mentoring	R = reports/documentation
B = lunch/break	O = other	

Note. Practitioner duties differ from district to district; the above list should be edited accordingly.

6

Supervision of Occupational Therapy Assistants in Schools

Supervision of occupational therapy service delivery is a collaborative process between supervisors and supervisees. The American Occupational Therapy Association's (AOTA's; 2014a) *Guidelines for Supervision, Roles, and Responsibilities During the Delivery of Occupational Therapy Services* (available in Appendix D) identify two purposes of supervision:

1. To ensure "the safe and effective delivery of occupational therapy services" and
2. To foster "professional competence and development" (p. S16).

The delivery of occupational therapy services is guided by AOTA's official documents and regulated in all 50 states, the District of Colombia, and Puerto Rico (AOTA, 2014b). Regulations for the supervision of occupational therapy services vary from state to state. Occupational therapy practitioners must understand and follow all relevant requirements for supervision and the documentation of supervisory activities within their state. A state-by-state listing of the statutes and regulations related to supervision is provided on the AOTA website (http://bit.ly/2l0tSv2).

ENSURING SAFE AND EFFECTIVE OCCUPATIONAL THERAPY

Once occupational therapists have received the appropriate education, credentials, and licensure, they are able to practice autonomously and are ultimately responsible for all aspects of the occupational therapy process (AOTA, 2015). An occupational therapy assistant, however, must provide services under the supervision of and in collaboration with an occupational therapist (AOTA, 2014a). In general, occupational therapy assistants are responsible for demonstrating service competency and seeking out the supervision they need to provide safe and effective occupational therapy services, whereas the occupational therapist is responsible for delegating tasks appropriately and for providing an appropriate level of supervision (AOTA, 2014a). Services delegated to an occupational therapy assistant should be documented on the occupational therapy intervention plan (see Chapter 4, "Intervention: Planning, Implementation, and Review").

The methods used for supervision, how often the supervision is provided, and the topics covered during supervision contacts differ depending on a variety of factors, including the needs of the clients, the skills and expertise of the occupational therapist and occupational therapy assistant, the characteristics of the client population and practice setting,

the institution's policies, and state regulations (AOTA, 2014a). Table 6.1 provides an overview of the roles and responsibilities of occupational therapists and occupational therapy assistants throughout the occupational therapy process as described in *Guidelines for Supervision, Roles, and Responsibilities During the Delivery of Occupational Therapy Services* (AOTA, 2014a).

Supervision can be provided using direct, face-to-face interactions (e.g., observation, modeling, discussion, training, video conferencing) or indirect interactions (e.g., phone contacts, email, written communication; AOTA 2014a). Jost and Rohn (2013) recommended that both the occupational therapist and the occupational therapy assistant sign and maintain copies of any documentation related to supervision.

When documenting the plan for supervision and supervision contacts, the occupational therapist and occupational therapy assistant must follow the procedures required state regulations and school district policies (AOTA, 2014a). *Guidelines for Supervision, Roles, and Responsibilities During the Delivery of Occupational Therapy Services*

Table 6.1   OVERVIEW OF THE ROLES OF OCCUPATIONAL THERAPIST AND OCCUPATIONAL THERAPY ASSISTANT

OCCUPATIONAL THERAPY PROCESS	OCCUPATIONAL THERAPIST	OCCUPATIONAL THERAPY ASSISTANT
Evaluation (or screening)	Initiates and directs the evaluation or screening process, interprets data, determines need for services, identifies goals or priorities, delegates specific tasks to the OTA as appropriate, interprets information gathered by the OTA, and incorporates it into the evaluation.	Contributes to the evaluation or screening process by carrying out delegated tasks and reporting to the OT; does not make decisions about the need for OT services.
Intervention Planning	Develops occupational therapy intervention plan in collaboration with the OTA and client.	Is knowledgeable about the results of the evaluation; contributes to the intervention plan by providing input to the OT.
Intervention Implementation	Takes responsibility for implementing occupational therapy interventions, delegates aspects of occupational therapy intervention to the OTA, and provides appropriate supervision.	Is knowledgeable about the client's occupational therapy goals; collaborates with the OT to select, implement, and modify interventions.
Intervention Review	Determines whether to continue, modify, or discontinue occupational therapy services.	Supports intervention review by providing the OT with information and documentation related to client responses during occupational therapy sessions.
Targeting and Evaluating Outcomes	Selects, measures, and interprets outcomes related to client engagement in occupations.	Is knowledgeable about identified outcomes for the client; provides the OT with information and documentation related to achievement of outcomes.
Documentation	Follows the procedures for documenting a plan for supervision and supervision contacts as required by school district policies and state regulations.	Follows the procedures for documenting a plan for supervision and supervision contacts as required by state regulations and school district policies.

Note. OT = occupational therapist; OTA = occupational therapy assistant.
Source. AOTA (2014a).

(AOTA, 2014a) provides the following list that could be included when documenting supervision:

- Frequency of supervisory contact,
- Methods or types of supervision,
- Content areas addressed,
- Evidence to support areas and levels of competency, and
- Names and credentials of the persons participating in the supervisory process (pp. S17–S18).

Form 6.A, "Sample OT and OTA Collaboration/Supervision Record," provides an example of a supervision record that is used collaboratively by the occupational therapist and occupational therapy assistant. The date, time, topic (or students) discussed, and the plan are entered each time the occupational therapist and occupational therapy assistant meet. Both sign it at the bottom and keep a copy for their records. If there is more than one supervising occupational therapist, they may choose to share this form or each have their own form.

SUPERVISION TO SUPPORT PROFESSIONAL GROWTH

Professional growth is critical for maintaining competence for occupational therapy practitioners, and the occupational therapist should support professional development and goal setting for the occupational therapy assistant. Development of professional goals may include learning a new technique, gathering more background on a specific medical diagnosis, or studying systematic reviews on interventions for facilitating self-care skills.

After the practitioner identifies goals, an action plan is developed that lists the steps needed to achieve the goal, estimated timelines to achieve the step, and a description of how to determine the goal has been met. The action plan can be documented in Form 6.B, "Professional Development Plan for OTAs." This plan is reviewed periodically to determine progress toward the goal.

SUMMARY

Occupational therapists and occupational therapy assistants have a joint responsibility for ensuring safe and effective occupational therapy services and for maintaining appropriate documentation of supervision contacts.

REFERENCES

American Occupational Therapy Association. (2014a). Guidelines for supervision, roles, and responsibilities during the delivery of occupational therapy services. *American Journal of Occupational Therapy, 68*(Suppl. 3), S16–S22. https://doi.org/10.5014/ajot.2014.686S03

American Occupational Therapy Association. (2014b). *Jurisdictions regulating occupational therapy*. Retrieved from http://www.aota.org/advocacy-policy/state-policy/licensure/stateregs/jurisdictions-regulating-occupational-therapists.aspx

American Occupational Therapy Association. (2015). Standards of practice for occupational therapy. *American Journal of Occupational Therapy, 69*(Suppl. 3), 1–6. https://doi.org/10.5014/ajot.2015.696S06

FORM 6.A. SAMPLE OT AND OTA COLLABORATION/SUPERVISION RECORD

OT AND OTA COLLABORATION/SUPERVISION RECORD

Month: _____   Year: _____

OTA Name: _____

Supervising OT(s): _____

Directions: Complete. Each OT and OTA should keep a copy for their records.

Date and Time	Topics or Students Discussed	Plan (Changes to Intervention or Other Decisions)

Signature of OTA: _____   Date _____

Signature of Supervising OT: _____   Date _____

Note. OT = occupational therapist; OTA = occupational therapy assistant.

FORM 6.B. PROFESSIONAL DEVELOPMENT PLAN FOR OTAs

Professional Development Plan for Academic Year: _____

Name:	
Goal:	
Reason for choosing this goal:	

Action Plan

List Action Steps You Will Take to Achieve Goal	List Timelines to Complete This Step	Describe How You Know This Step Is Met (e.g., Evidence, Outcome)

Review of Plan

OTA Signature: _____   Date: _____

Supervising OT Signature: _____   Date: _____

Note. OT = occupational therapist; OTA = occupational therapy assistant.

Documentation for
Medicaid Services in Schools

Many public schools and educational agencies bill the state Medicaid program to recoup some of their costs in providing services required under the Individuals with Disabilities Education Improvement Act of 2004 (IDEA; P. L. 108–446). The Medicaid program is a primary payer for students who are eligible for Medicaid and receive direct covered services under Part B of IDEA (Medicare Catastrophic Coverage Act of 1988; P. L. 100–360). Practitioners are accountable for services they provide and must be educated about billing and reimbursement policies. Occupational therapy practitioners are bound by the *Occupational Therapy Code of Ethics (2015)* (American Occupational Therapy Association [AOTA], 2015), which requires practitioners to take responsibility for billing their services and educating administrators about their ethical obligations (Frolek Clark & Holahan, 2015).

BILLING MEDICAID

In compliance with federal and state Medicaid policy, occupational therapy practitioners working in schools may bill Medicaid for services when
- Signed parental consent has been provided;
- Services are medically necessary as defined by the state Medicaid plan or an agreement between the state Medicaid agency and the state education agency;
- Services are coverable under a federal Medicaid coverage category;
- All federal and state regulations, including those for provider qualifications and other requirements, have been followed; and

- Services are included as covered services in the state plan or are required to be covered under the requirements of the early periodic screening, diagnosis, and treatment mandate (Centers for Medicare and Medicaid Services [CMS], 2003).

On the basis of state Medicaid policy, occupational therapy screenings and evaluations may be covered for students who are eligible for Medicaid if the services meet the above criteria for Medicaid reimbursement. Also, billing must comply with federal and state policy.

In some states, under the state Medicaid plan or other agreements, medical necessity may require a physician's referral or signature. Other states may consider a student's individualized education program (IEP) team process as sufficient for proving medical necessity, allowing reimbursement of occupational therapy services if they are listed on the IEP. There is no inherent conflict between services included in an IEP to support access to the curriculum and medical necessity; states address this through their own policies.

EVALUATION CODING

New evaluation codes for occupational therapy evaluations were instituted January 1, 2017, in the *Common Procedure Terminology® (CPT)* owned and produced by the American Medical Association. Three new codes must be used for evaluation (97165, 97166, 97167) that are based on the complexity of the evaluation (low, moderate, very complex). There is also a new reevaluation code (97168).

Definitions of the new evaluation codes provide solid direction for an optimal occupational therapy evaluation based on principles of the *Occupational Therapy Practice Framework: Domain and Process* (AOTA, 2014). According to the code language, occupational therapy evaluations must include an occupational profile (see Appendix F, "AOTA Occupational Profile Template") and review of medical and therapy history and assessment. Further, the codes support occupational therapy's review of physical, cognitive, and psychosocial skills, appropriately validating the full scope of occupational therapy practice. Medicaid agencies will be required to use these new codes in billing, so therapists must become familiar with the new descriptions. For basic resources on these new codes, see Appendix G, "New Occupational Therapy Evaluation Coding Overview."

These codes recognize the full scope of the occupational therapy profession and are a new opportunity to describe and implement occupational therapy. Although the codes may be used only sometimes in school-based practice, all occupational therapists and occupational therapy assistants should understand the principles and language of the new codes.

The definition of *evaluation* and *reevaluation* under IDEA may be somewhat different from the *CPT* definitions. The occupational therapy evaluation determines the need for service and the development of a plan of care. However, under IDEA, the term *evaluation* is typically used to identify the initial evaluation, which occurs before any special education and related services can be provided.

States and districts may also define *reevaluation* in different ways. Each state and some school districts have guidance on how services are defined and when and how to use the codes for billing Medicaid or other documentation. Readers should review and understand their state and district policies and definitions for billing Medicaid and other reporting requirements.

OTHER BILLING REQUIREMENTS

Beyond understanding the new evaluation codes and knowing when to appropriately use them in school settings and for billing Medicaid, practitioners must understand other requirements for billing Medicaid:

- Occupational therapy services must be provided with the student present (e.g., not during IEP or teacher meetings) to receive reimbursement from Medicaid.
- If students are seen in a group, the group billing *CPT* or other code must be used.
- Date and time must be documented (some states require specific recording of time in and time out).
- Interventions must be related to the student's medical condition or disability.
- Service contact logs and progress notes must provide the date, length of intervention session, location of service, the skilled interventions used, information about the student, and any medical documentation related to the medical condition or diagnosis (CMS, 1997).

Although documentation forms are state- and school-specific, the following resources (in addition to Appendixes F and G) may assist occupational therapy practitioners when completing these forms:

- "Medicaid FAQ for School Occupational Therapy Practitioners" (Frolek Clark & Holahan, 2015)
- "School Systems FAQ" (AOTA, n.d.).

REFERENCES

American Medical Association. (2017). *CPT 2017: Professional edition*. Chicago: Author.

American Occupational Therapy Association. (2014). Occupational therapy practice framework: Domain and process. *American Journal of Occupational Therapy, 68*(Suppl. 1), S1–S48. https://10.5014/ajot/2014.682006

American Occupational Therapy Association (2015). Occupational therapy code of ethics. *American Journal of Occupational Therapy, 69*(6 Suppl.), 6913410030. https://doi.org/10.5014/ajot.2010.64S17

American Occupational Therapy Association. (2017). *AOTA Occupational profile template.* Retrieved from https://www.aota.org/~/media/Corporate/Files/Practice/Manage/Documentation/AOTA-Occupational-Profile-Template.pdf

American Occupational Therapy Association. (n.d.). *School systems FAQ.* Retrieved from http://www.aota.org/Advocacy-Policy/Federal-Reg-Affairs/Pay/Schools/School-System.aspx

Centers for Medicare and Medicaid Services (1997). *Medicaid and school health: A technical assistance guide.* Retrieved from https://www.medicaid.gov/medicaid/financingand reimbursement/downloads/school_based_user_guide.pdf

Centers for Medicare and Medicaid Services. (2003). *Medicaid school-based administrative claiming guide.* Retrieved from https://www.cms.gov/research-statistics-data-and-systems/computer-data-and-systems/medicaidbudgetexpendsystem/downloads/schoolhealthsvcs.pdf

Frolek Clark, G. & Holahan, L. (2015). Medicaid FAQ for school occupational therapy practitioners. *OT Practice, 20*(20), 18–24.

Individuals with Disabilities Education Improvement Act of 2004, Pub. L. 108–446, 20 U.S.C. §1400 et seq.

Medicare Catastrophic Coverage Act of 1988, Pub. L. 100–360, 102 Stat. 683.

Appendix A.
Guidelines for Documentation of Occupational Therapy

Documentation of occupational therapy services is necessary whenever professional services are provided to a client. Occupational therapists and occupational therapy assistants[1] determine the appropriate type of documentation structure and then record the services provided within their scope of practice. This document, based on the *Occupational Therapy Practice Framework: Domain and Process* (2nd ed.; American Occupational Therapy Association [AOTA], 2008), describes the components and purpose of professional documentation used in occupational therapy.

AOTA's (2010) *Standards of Practice for Occupational Therapy* states that an occupational therapy practitioner[2] documents the occupational therapy services and "abides by the time frames, format, and standards established by the practice settings, government agencies, external accreditation programs, payers, and AOTA documents" (p. S108). These requirements apply to both electronic and written forms of documentation. Documentation should reflect the nature of services provided and the clinical reasoning of the occupational therapy practitioner, and it should provide enough information to ensure that services are delivered in a safe and effective manner. Documentation should describe the depth and breadth of services provided to meet the complexity of individual client[3] needs. The client's diagnosis or prognosis should not be used as the sole rationale for occupational therapy services.

The purpose of documentation is to

- Communicate information about the client from the occupational therapy perspective;

- Articulate the rationale for provision of occupational therapy services and the relationship of those services to client outcomes, reflecting the occupational therapy practitioner's clinical reasoning and professional judgment; and

- Create a chronological record of client status, occupational therapy services provided to the client, client response to occupational therapy intervention, and client outcomes.

Types of Documentation

Table 1 outlines common types of documentation reports. Reports may be named differently or combined and reorganized to meet the specific needs of the setting. Occupational therapy documentation should always record the practitioner's activity in the areas of screening, evaluation, intervention, and outcomes (AOTA, 2008) in accordance with payer, facility, and state and federal guidelines.

---

[1]*Occupational therapists* are responsible for all aspects of occupational therapy service delivery and are accountable for the safety and effectiveness of the occupational therapy service delivery process. *Occupational therapy assistants* deliver occupational therapy services under the supervision of and in partnership with an occupational therapist (AOTA, 2009).

[2]When the term *occupational therapy practitioner* is used in this document, it refers to both occupational therapists and occupational therapy assistants (AOTA, 2006).

[3]In this document, *client* may refer to an individual, organization, or population.

Table 1. Common Types of Occupational Therapy Documentation Reports

Process Areas	Type of Report
I. Screening	A. Screening Report
II. Evaluation	A. Evaluation Report
	B. Reevaluation Report
III. Intervention	A. Intervention Plan
	B. Contact Report Note or Communiqué
	C. Progress Report/Note
	D. Transition Plan
IV. Outcomes	A. Discharge/Discontinuation Report

Content of Reports

I. Screening

    A. Documents referral source, reason for occupational therapy screening, and need for occupational therapy evaluation and service.

        1. Phone referrals should be documented in accordance with payer, facility, and state and federal guidelines and include

            a. Names of individuals spoken with,

            b. Purpose of screening,

            c. Date of request,

            d. Number of contact for referral source, and

            e. Description of client's prior level of occupational performance.

    B. Consists of an initial brief assessment to determine client's need for an occupational therapy evaluation or for referral to another service if not appropriate for occupational therapy services.

    C. Suggested content:

        1. *Client information*—Name/agency; date of birth; gender; health status; and applicable medical/educational/developmental diagnoses, precautions, and contraindications

        2. *Referral information*—Date and source of referral, services requested, reason for referral, funding source, and anticipated length of service

        3. *Brief occupational profile*—Client's reason for seeking occupational therapy services, current areas of occupation that are successful and problematic, contexts and environments that support and hinder occupations, medical/educational/work history, occupational history (e.g., patterns of living, interest, values), client's priorities, and targeted goals

        4. *Assessments used and results*—Types of assessments used and results (e.g., interviews, record reviews, observations)

        5. *Recommendation*—Professional judgments regarding appropriateness of need for complete occupational therapy evaluation.

II. Evaluation

A. Evaluation Report

   1. Documents referral source and data gathered through the evaluation process in accordance with payer, facility, state, and/or federal guidelines. Includes

      a. Analysis of occupational performance and identification of factors that support and hinder performance and participation and

      b. Identification of specific areas of occupation and occupational performance to be addressed, interventions, and expected outcomes.

   2. Suggested content:

      a. *Client information*—Name; date of birth; gender; health status; medical history; and applicable medical/educational/developmental diagnoses, precautions, and contraindications

      b. *Referral information*—Date and source of referral, services requested, reason for referral, funding source, and anticipated length of service

      c. *Occupational profile*—Client's reason for seeking occupational therapy services, current areas of occupation that are successful and problematic, contexts and environments that support or hinder occupations, medical/educational/work history, occupational history (e.g., patterns of living, interest, values), client's priorities, and targeted outcomes

      d. *Assessments used and results*—Types of assessments used and results (e.g., interviews, record reviews, observations, standardized and/or nonstandardized assessments)

      e. *Analysis of occupational performance*—Description of and judgment about performance skills, performance patterns, contexts and environments, activity demands, outcomes from standardized measures and/or nonstandardized assessments,[4] and client factors that will be targeted for intervention and outcomes expected

      f. *Summary and analysis*—Interpretation and summary of data as related to occupational profile and referring concern

      g. *Recommendation*—Judgment regarding appropriateness of occupational therapy services or other services.

      Note. The intervention plan, including intervention goals addressing anticipated outcomes, objectives, and frequency of therapy, is described in the "Intervention Plan" section that follows.

B. Reevaluation Report

   1. Documents the results of the reevaluation process. Frequency of reevaluation depends on the needs of the setting, the progress of the client, and client changes.

   2. Suggested content:

      a. *Client information*—Name; date of birth; gender; and applicable medical/educational/developmental diagnoses, precautions, and contraindications

      b. *Occupational profile*—Updates on current areas of occupation that are successful and problematic, contexts and environments that support or hinder occupations, summary of any new medical/educational/work information, and updates or changes to client's priorities and targeted outcomes

---

[4]*Nonstandardized assessment tools* are considered a valid form of information gathering that allows for flexibility and individualization when measuring outcomes related to the status of an individual or group through an intrapersonal comparison. Although not uniform in administration or scoring or possessing full and complete psychometric data, nonstandardized assessment tools possess strong internal validity and represent an evidence-based approach to occupational therapy practice (Hinojosa, Kramer, & Crist, 2010). Nonstandardized tools should be selected on the basis of the best available evidence and the clinical reasoning of the practitioner.

c. *Reevaluation results*—Focus of reevaluation, specific types of outcome measures from standardized and/or nonstandardized assessments used, and client's performance and subjective responses

d. *Analysis of occupational performance*—Description of and judgment about performance skills, performance patterns, contexts and environments, activity demands, outcomes from standardized measures and/or nonstandardized assessments, and client factors that will be targeted for intervention and outcomes expected

e. *Summary and analysis*—Interpretation and summary of data as related to referring concern and comparison of results with previous evaluation results

f. *Recommendations*—Changes to occupational therapy services, revision or continuation of interventions, goals and objectives, frequency of occupational therapy services, and recommendation for referral to other professionals or agencies as applicable.

III. Intervention

A. Intervention Plan

1. Documents the goals, intervention approaches, and types of interventions to be used to achieve the client's identified targeted outcomes and is based on results of evaluation or reevaluation processes. Includes recommendations or referrals to other professionals and agencies in adherence with each payer source documentation requirements (e.g., pain levels, time spent on each modality).

2. Suggested content:

a. *Client information*—Name, date of birth, gender, precautions, and contraindications

b. *Intervention goals*—Measurable and meaningful occupation-based long-term and short-term objective goals directly related to the client's ability and need to engage in desired occupations

c. *Intervention approaches and types of interventions to be used*—Intervention approaches that include create/promote, establish/restore, maintain, modify, and/or prevent; types of interventions that include consultation, education process, advocacy, and/or the therapeutic use of occupations or activities

d. *Service delivery mechanisms*—Service provider, service location, and frequency and duration of services

e. *Plan for discharge*—Discontinuation criteria, discharge setting (e.g., skilled nursing facility, home, community, classroom) and follow-up care

f. *Outcome measures*—Tools that assess occupational performance, adaptation, role competence, improved health and wellness, improved quality of life, self-advocacy, and occupational justice. Standardized and/or nonstandardized assessments used at evaluation should be readministered periodically to monitor measurable progress and report functional outcomes as required by client's payer source and/or facility requirements.

g. *Professionals responsible and date of plan*—Names and positions of persons overseeing plan, date plan was developed, and date when plan was modified or reviewed.

B. Service Contacts

1. Documents contacts between the client and the occupational therapy practitioner. Records the types of interventions used and client's response, which can include telephone contacts, interventions, and meetings with others.

2. Suggested content:

a. *Client information*—Name; date of birth; gender; and diagnosis, precautions, and contraindications

b. *Therapy log*—Date, type of contact, names/positions of persons involved, summary or significant information communicated during contacts, client attendance and participation in intervention, reason service is missed, types of interventions used, client's response, environmental or task modification, assistive or adaptive devices used or fabricated, statement of any training education or consultation provided, and the client's present level of performance. Documentation of services provided should reflect the complexity of the client and the professional clinical reasoning and expertise of an occupational therapy practitioner required to provide an effective outcome in occupational performance. The client's diagnosis or prognosis should not be the sole rationale for the skilled interventions provided. Measures used to assess outcomes should be repeated in accordance with payer and facility requirements and documented to demonstrate measurable functional progress of the client.

   c. *Intervention/procedure coding* (i.e., *CPT™*),[5] if applicable.

C. Progress Report/Note

   1. Summarizes intervention process and documents client's progress toward achievement of goals. Includes new data collected; modifications of treatment plan; and statement of need for continuation, discontinuation, or referral.

   2. Suggested content:

      a. *Client information*—Name; date of birth; gender; and diagnosis, precautions, and contraindications

      b. *Summary of services provided*—Brief statement of frequency of services and length of time services have been provided; techniques and strategies used; measurable progress or lack thereof using age-appropriate current functional standardized and/or nonstandardized outcome measures; environmental or task modifications provided; adaptive equipment or orthotics provided; medical, educational, or other pertinent client updates; client's response to occupational therapy services; and programs or training provided to the client or caregivers

      c. *Current client performance*—Client's progress toward the goals and client's performance in areas of occupations

      d. *Plan or recommendations*—Recommendations and rationale as well as client's input to changes or continuation of plan.

D. Transition Plan

   1. Documents the formal transition plan and is written when client is transitioning from one service setting to another within a service delivery system.

   2. Suggested content:

      a. *Client information*—Name; date of birth; gender; and diagnosis, precautions, and contraindications

      b. *Client's current status*—Client's current performance in occupations

      c. *Transition plan*—Name of current service setting and name of setting to which client will transition, reason for transition, time frame in which transition will occur, and outline of activities to be carried out during the transition plan

      d. *Recommendations*—Recommendations and rationale for occupational therapy services, modifications or accommodations needed, and assistive technology and environmental modifications needed.

IV. Outcomes

A. Discharge Report—Summary of Occupational Therapy Services and Outcomes

   1. Summarizes the changes in client's ability to engage in occupations between the initial evaluation and discontinuation of services and makes recommendations as applicable.

   2. Suggested content with examples include

      a. *Client information*—name/agency, date of birth, gender, diagnosis, precautions, and contraindications

---

[5]*CPT* is a trademark of the American Medical Association (AMA). *CPT* five-digit codes, nomenclature, and other data are copyright © 2011 by the AMA. All rights reserved.

Box 1. Fundamentals of Documentation

- Client's full name and case number (if applicable) on each page of documentation
- Date
- Identification of type of documentation (e.g., evaluation report, progress report/note)
- Occupational therapy practitioner's signature with a minimum of first name or initial, last name, and professional designation
- When applicable, signature of the recorder directly after the documentation entry. If additional information is needed, a signed addendum must be added to the record.
- Cosignature of an occupational therapist or occupational therapy assistant on student documentation, as required by payer policy, governing laws and regulations, and/or employer
- Compliance with all laws, regulations, payer, and employer requirements
- Acceptable terminology defined within the boundaries of setting
- Abbreviations usage as acceptable within the boundaries of setting
- All errors noted and signed
- Adherence to professional standards of technology, when used to document occupational therapy services with electronic claims or records.
- Disposal of records (electronic and traditionally written) within law or agency requirements
- Compliance with confidentiality standards
- Compliance with agency or legal requirements of storage of records
- Documentation should reflect professional clinical reasoning and expertise of an occupational therapy practitioner and the nature of occupational therapy services delivered in a safe and effective manner. The client's diagnosis or prognosis should not be the sole rationale for occupational therapy services.

    b. *Summary of intervention process*—date of initial and final service; frequency, number of sessions, summary of interventions used; summary of progress toward goals; and occupational therapy outcomes—initial client status and ending status regarding engagement in occupations, client's assessment of efficacy of occupational therapy services

    c. *Recommendations*—recommendations pertaining to the client's future needs; specific follow-up plans, if applicable; and referrals to other professionals and agencies, if applicable.

Each occupational therapy client has a client record maintained as a permanent file. The record is maintained in a professional and legal fashion (i.e., organized, legible, concise, clear, accurate, complete, current, grammatically correct, and objective; see Box 1 for more information).

References

American Medical Association. (2011). *Current procedural terminology.* Chicago: Author.

American Occupational Therapy Association. (2006). Policy 1.41. Categories of occupational therapy personnel. In *Policy manual* (2011 ed.). Bethesda, MD: Author.

American Occupational Therapy Association. (2008). Occupational therapy practice framework: Domain and process (2nd ed.). *American Journal of Occupational Therapy, 62,* 625–683. http://dx.doi.org/10.5014/ajot.62.6.625

American Occupational Therapy Association. (2009). Guidelines for supervision, roles, and responsibilities during the delivery of occupational therapy services. *American Journal of Occupational Therapy, 63,* 797–803. http://dx.doi.org/10.5014/ajot.63.6.797

American Occupational Therapy Association. (2010). Standards of practice for occupational therapy. *American Journal of Occupational Therapy, 64*(Suppl.), S106–S111. http://dx.doi.org/10.5014/ajot.2010.64S106

Hinojosa, J., Kramer, P., & Crist, P. (2010). *Evaluation: Obtaining and interpreting data* (3rd ed.). Bethesda, MD: AOTA Press.

Authors

Gloria Frolek Clark, MS, OTR/L, FAOTA
Mary Jane Youngstrom, MS, OTR/L, FAOTA

for

The Commission on Practice
Sara Jane Brayman, PhD, OTR/L, FAOTA, *Chairperson*

Adopted by the Representative Assembly 2003M16

Edited by the Commission on Practice 2007

Edited by the Commission on Practice 2012
Debbie Amini, EdD, OTR/L, CHT, *Chairperson*

Adopted by the Representative Assembly Coordinating Council (RACC) for the Representative Assembly, 2012

Note. This revision replaces the 2007 document previously published and copyrighted in 2008 by the American Occupational Therapy Association in the *American Journal of Occupational Therapy, 62,* 684–690.

Citation. American Occupational Therapy Association. (2013). Guidelines for documentation of occupational therapy. *American Journal of Occupational Therapy, 67*(Suppl.), S32–S38. http://doi.org/10.5014/ajot.62.6.684

Appendix B.
Standards of Practice for Occupational Therapy

This document defines minimum standards for the practice of occupational therapy. The *practice of occupational therapy* means the therapeutic use of occupations (everyday life activities) with persons, groups, and populations for the purpose of participation in roles and situations in the home, school, workplace, community, or other settings.

Occupational therapy services are provided for habilitation, rehabilitation, and the promotion of health and wellness to those who have or are at risk for developing an illness, injury, disease, disorder, condition, impairment, disability, activity limitation, or participation restriction. Occupational therapy addresses the physical, cognitive, psychosocial, sensory–perceptual, and other aspects of performance in a variety of contexts and environments to support engagement in occupations that affect physical and mental health, well-being, and quality of life (American Occupational Therapy Association [AOTA], 2011). The overarching goal of occupational therapy is to support people in participation in life through engagement in occupation for "habilitation, rehabilitation, and promotion of health and wellness for clients with disability- and non–disability-related needs" (AOTA, 2014b, p. S1).

The *Standards of Practice for Occupational Therapy* are requirements for occupational therapists and occupational therapy assistants for the delivery of occupational therapy services. *The Reference Manual of the Official Documents of the American Occupational Therapy Association, Inc.* (AOTA, 2015b) contains documents that clarify and support occupational therapy practice, as do various issues of the *American Journal of Occupational Therapy.* These documents are reviewed and updated on an ongoing basis for their applicability.

Education, Examination, and Licensure Requirements

All occupational therapists and occupational therapy assistants must practice under federal and state laws. To practice as an occupational therapist, the individual must

- Have graduated from an occupational therapy program accredited by the Accreditation Council for Occupational Therapy Education (ACOTE®) or predecessor organizations;

- Have successfully completed a period of supervised fieldwork experience required by the recognized educational institution where the applicant met the academic requirements of an educational program for occupational therapists that is accredited by ACOTE or predecessor organizations;

- Have passed the entry-level examination for occupational therapists approved by the state occupational therapy regulatory board or agency; and

- Fulfill state requirements for licensure, certification, or registration. Internationally educated occupational therapists must complete occupational therapy education programs (including fieldwork requirements) that are deemed comparable (by the credentialing body recognized by the state occupational therapy regulatory board or agency) to entry-level occupational therapy education programs in the United States.

To practice as an occupational therapy assistant, the individual must

- Have graduated from an occupational therapy assistant program accredited by ACOTE or predecessor organizations;
- Have successfully completed a period of supervised fieldwork experience required by the recognized educational institution where the applicant met the academic requirements of an educational program for occupational therapy assistants that is accredited by ACOTE or predecessor organizations;
- Have passed the entry-level examination for occupational therapy assistants approved by the state occupational therapy regulatory board or agency; and
- Fulfill state requirements for licensure, certification, or registration.

Definitions

The following definitions are used in this document. All definitions are retrieved from the *Occupational Therapy Practice Framework: Domain and Process* (AOTA, 2014b) unless noted otherwise:

- *Activities:* Actions designed and selected to support the development of performance skills and performance patterns to enhance occupational engagement (AOTA, 2014b, p. S41).
- *Assessments:* "Specific tools or instruments that are used during the evaluation process" (AOTA, 2010, p. S107).
- *Client:* Person or persons (including those involved in the care of a client), group (collective of individuals, e.g., families, workers, students, or community members), or population (collective of groups or individuals living in a similar locale—e.g., city, state, or country—or sharing the same or like concerns) (AOTA, 2014b, p. S41).
- *Evaluation:* "Process of obtaining and interpreting data necessary for intervention. This includes planning for and documenting the evaluation process and results" (AOTA, 2010, p. S107).
- *Intervention:* "Process and skilled actions taken by occupational therapy practitioners in collaboration with the client to facilitate engagement in occupation related to health and participation. The intervention process includes the plan, implementation, and review" (AOTA, 2010, p. S107; see Table 6).
- *Occupation*: Daily life activities in which people engage. Occupations occur in context and are influenced by the interplay among client factors, performance skills, and performance patterns. Occupations occur over time; have purpose, meaning, and perceived utility to the client; and can be observed by others (e.g., preparing a meal) or be known only to the person involved (e.g., learning through reading a textbook). Occupations can involve the execution of multiple activities for completion and can result in various outcomes. The *Framework* identifies a broad range of occupations categorized as activities of daily living, instrumental activities of daily living, rest and sleep, education, work, play, leisure, and social participation (AOTA, 2014b, p. S43).
- *Outcome:* End result of the occupational therapy process; what clients can achieve through occupational therapy intervention (AOTA, 2014b, p. S44).
- *Reevaluation*: Reappraisal of the client's performance and goals to determine the type and amount of change that has taken place (AOTA, 2014b, p. S45).
- *Screening:* Obtaining and reviewing data relevant to a potential client to determine the need for further evaluation and intervention.
- *Transitions*: Actions coordinated to prepare for or facilitate a change, such as from one functional level to another, from one life [change] to another, from one program to another, or from one environment to another.

Standard I. Professional Standing and Responsibility

1. An occupational therapy practitioner (occupational therapist or occupational therapy assistant) delivers occupational therapy services that reflect the philosophical base of occupational therapy and are consistent with the established principles and concepts of theory and practice.

2. An occupational therapy practitioner is knowledgeable about and delivers occupational therapy services in accordance with AOTA standards, policies, and guidelines and state, federal, and other regulatory and payer requirements relevant to practice and service delivery.

3. An occupational therapy practitioner maintains current licensure, registration, or certification as required by law or regulation.

4. An occupational therapy practitioner abides by the *Occupational Therapy Code of Ethics (2015)* (AOTA, 2015a).

5. An occupational therapy practitioner abides by the *Standards for Continuing Competence* (AOTA, 2015c) by establishing, maintaining, and updating professional performance, knowledge, and skills.

6. An occupational therapist is responsible for all aspects of occupational therapy service delivery and is accountable for the safety and effectiveness of the occupational therapy service delivery process (AOTA, 2014a).

7. An occupational therapy assistant is responsible for providing safe and effective occupational therapy services under the "direct and indirect" supervision of and in partnership with the occupational therapist and in accordance with laws or regulations and AOTA documents (AOTA, 2014a).

8. An occupational therapy practitioner maintains current knowledge of legislative, political, social, cultural, societal, and reimbursement issues that affect clients and the practice of occupational therapy.

9. An occupational therapy practitioner is knowledgeable about evidence-based practice and applies it ethically and appropriately to provide occupational therapy services consistent with best practice approaches.

10. An occupational therapy practitioner obtains the client's consent throughout the occupational therapy process.

11. An occupational therapy practitioner is an effective advocate for the client's intervention and/or accommodation needs.

12. An occupational therapy practitioner is an integral member of the interdisciplinary collaborative health care team. He or she consults with team and family members to ensure the client-centeredness of evaluation and intervention practices.

13. An occupational therapy practitioner respects the client's sociocultural background and provides client-centered and family-centered occupational therapy services.

Standard II. Screening, Evaluation, and Reevaluation

1. An occupational therapist is responsible for all aspects of the screening, evaluation, and reevaluation process.

2. An occupational therapist accepts and responds to referrals in compliance with state or federal laws, other regulatory and payer requirements, and AOTA documents.

3. An occupational therapist, in collaboration with the client, evaluates the client's ability to participate in daily life tasks, roles, and responsibilities by considering the client's history, goals, capacities, and needs; analysis of task components; the activities and occupations the client wants and needs to perform; and the environments and context in which these activities and occupations occur.

4. An occupational therapist initiates and directs the screening, evaluation, and reevaluation process and analyzes and interprets the data in accordance with federal and state laws, other regulatory and payer requirements, and AOTA documents.

5. An occupational therapy assistant contributes to the screening, evaluation, and reevaluation process by administering delegated assessments and by providing verbal and written reports of observations and client capacities to the occupational therapist in accordance with federal and state laws, other regulatory and payer requirements, and AOTA documents.

6. An occupational therapy practitioner uses current assessments and assessment procedures and follows defined protocols of standardized assessments and needs assessment methods during the screening, evaluation, and reevaluation process.

7. An occupational therapist completes and documents the results of the occupational therapy evaluation. An occupational therapy assistant may contribute to the documentation of evaluation results. An occupational therapy practitioner abides by the time frames, formats, and standards established by practice settings, federal and state laws, other regulatory and payer requirements, external accreditation programs, and AOTA documents.

8. An occupational therapy practitioner communicates screening, evaluation, and reevaluation results within the boundaries of client confidentiality and privacy regulations to the appropriate person, group, or population.

9. An occupational therapist recommends additional consultations or refers clients to appropriate resources when the needs of the client can best be served by the expertise of other professionals or services.

10. An occupational therapy practitioner educates current and potential referral sources about the scope of occupational therapy services and the process of initiating occupational therapy services.

Standard III: Intervention Process

1. An occupational therapist has overall responsibility for the development, documentation, and implementation of the occupational therapy intervention plan based on the evaluation, client goals, best available evidence, and professional and clinical reasoning. When delegating aspects of the occupational therapy intervention to the occupational therapy assistant, the occupational therapist is responsible for providing appropriate supervision.

2. An occupational therapist ensures that the intervention plan is documented within the time frames, formats, and standards established by the practice settings, agencies, external accreditation programs, state and federal laws, and other regulatory and payer requirements.

3. An occupational therapy practitioner collaborates with the client to develop and implement the intervention plan, on the basis of the client's needs and priorities, safety issues, and relative benefits and risks of the interventions and service delivery.

4. An occupational therapy practitioner coordinates the development and implementation of the occupational therapy intervention with the intervention provided by other professionals, when appropriate.

5. An occupational therapy practitioner uses professional and clinical reasoning, available evidence-based practice, and therapeutic use of self to select and implement the most appropriate types of interventions. Preparatory methods and tasks, education and training, advocacy, and group interventions are used, with meaningful occupations as the primary treatment modality, both as an ends and a means.

6. An occupational therapy assistant selects, implements, and makes modifications to therapeutic interventions that are consistent with the occupational therapy assistant's demonstrated competency and delegated responsibilities, the intervention plan, and requirements of the practice setting.

7. An occupational therapist modifies the intervention plan throughout the intervention process and documents changes in the client's needs, goals, and performance.

8. An occupational therapy assistant contributes to the modification of the intervention plan by exchanging information with and providing documentation to the occupational therapist about the client's responses to and communications throughout the intervention.

9. An occupational therapy practitioner documents the occupational therapy services provided within the time frames, formats, and standards established by the practice settings, agencies, external accreditation programs, federal and state laws, other regulatory and payer requirements, and AOTA documents.

Standard IV. Transition, Discharge, and Outcome Measurement

1. An occupational therapist is responsible for selecting, measuring, documenting, and interpreting expected and achieved outcomes that are related to the client's ability to engage in occupations.

2. An occupational therapist is responsible for documenting changes in the client's performance and capacities and for transitioning the client to other types or intensity of service or discontinuing services when the client has achieved identified goals, reached maximum benefit, or does not desire to continue services.

3. An occupational therapist prepares and implements a transition or discontinuation plan based on the client's needs, goals, performance, and appropriate follow-up resources.

4. An occupational therapy assistant contributes to the transition or discontinuation plan by providing information and documentation to the supervising occupational therapist related to the client's needs, goals, performance, and appropriate follow-up resources.

5. An occupational therapy practitioner facilitates the transition or discharge process in collaboration with the client, family members, significant others, other professionals (e.g., medical, educational, social services), and community resources, when appropriate.

6. An occupational therapist is responsible for evaluating the safety and effectiveness of the occupational therapy processes and interventions within the practice setting.

7. An occupational therapy assistant contributes to evaluating the safety and effectiveness of the occupational therapy processes and interventions within the practice setting.

8. The occupational therapy practitioner responsibly reports outcomes to payers and referring entities as well as to relevant local, regional, and national databases and registries, when appropriate.

References

American Occupational Therapy Association. (2010). Standards of practice for occupational therapy. *American Journal of Occupational Therapy, 64*(6, Suppl.), S106–S111. http://dx.doi.org/10.5014/ajot.2010.64S106

American Occupational Therapy Association. (2011). *Definition of occupational therapy practice for the AOTA Model Practice Act.* Retrieved from http://www.aota.org/-/media/Corporate/Files/Advocacy/State/Resources/PracticeAct/Model%20 Definition%20of%20OT%20Practice%20%20Adopted%2041411.ashx

American Occupational Therapy Association. (2014a). Guidelines for supervision, roles, and responsibilities during the delivery of occupational therapy services. *American Journal of Occupational Therapy, 68*(Suppl. 3), S16–S22. http://dx.doi.org/10.5014/ajot.2014.686S03

American Occupational Therapy Association. (2014b). Occupational therapy practice framework: Domain and process (3rd ed.). *American Journal of Occupational Therapy, 68*(Suppl. 1), S1–S48. http://dx.doi.org/10.5014/ajot.2014.682006

American Occupational Therapy Association. (2015a). Occupational therapy code of ethics (2015). *American Journal of Occupational Therapy, 69*(Suppl. 3), 6913410030. http://dx.doi.org/10.5014/ajot.2015.696S03

American Occupational Therapy Association. (2015b). *The reference manual of the official documents of the American Occupational Therapy Association, Inc.* (20th ed.). Bethesda, MD: AOTA Press.

American Occupational Therapy Association. (2015c). Standards for continuing competence. *American Journal of Occupational Therapy, 69*(Suppl. 3), 6913410055. http://dx.doi.org/10.5014/ajot.2015.696S16

Authors

Revised by the Commission on Practice, 2015:

Kathleen Kannenberg, MA, OTR/L, CCM, *Chairperson*

Salvador Bondoc, OTD, OTR/L, FAOTA

Cheryl Boop, MS, OTR/L

Meredith P. Gronski, OTD, OTR/L

Kimberly Kearney, COTA/L

Marsha Neville, PhD, OT

Janet M. Powell, PhD, OTR/L, FAOTA

Jerilyn (Gigi) Smith, PhD, OTR/L

Julie Dorsey, OTD, OTR/L, CEAS, *SIS Liaison*

Dottie Handley-More, MS, OTR/L, *Immediate-Past SIS Liaison*

Shannon Kelly, OT, *ASD Liaison*

Kiel Cooluris, MOT, OTR/L, *Immediate-Past ASD Liaison*

Deborah Lieberman, MHSA, OTR/L, FAOTA, *AOTA Headquarters Liaison*

For

The Commission on Practice
Kathleen Kannenberg, MA, OTR/L, CCM, *Chairperson*

The COP wishes to acknowledge the authors of the 2010 edition of this document: Janet V. DeLany, DEd, OTR/L, FAOTA, *Chairperson;* Debbie Amini, MEd, OTR/L, CHT; Ellen Cohn, ScD, OTR/L, FAOTA; Jennifer Cruz, MAT, MOTS, *ASD Liaison;* Kimberly Hartmann, PhD, OTR/L, FAOTA, *SISC Liaison;* Jeanette Justice, COTA/L; Kathleen Kannenberg, MA, OTR/L, CCM; Cherylin Lew, OTD, OTR/L; James Marc-Aurele, MBA, OTR/L; Mary Jane Youngstrom, MS, OTR, FAOTA; Deborah Lieberman, MHSA, OTR/L, FAOTA, *AOTA Headquarters Liaison*.

Adopted by the Representative Assembly, 2015NovCO14

Note. These standards are intended as recommended guidelines to assist occupational therapy practitioners in the provision of occupational therapy services. These standards serve as a minimum standard for occupational therapy practice and are applicable to all individual populations and the programs in which these individuals are served.

This revision replaces the 2010 document *Standards of Practice for Occupational Therapy* (previously published and copyrighted in 2010 by the American Occupational Therapy Association in the *American Journal of Occupational Therapy, 64*(Suppl.), S106–S111. http://dx.doi.org/10.5014/ajot.2010.64S106

Copyright © 2015 by the American Occupational Therapy Association. Reprinted with permission.

Citation. American Occupational Association. (2015). Standards of practice for occupational therapy. *American Journal of Occupational Therapy, 69*(Suppl. 3), 6913410057. http://dx.doi.org/10.5014/ajot.2015.696S06

Appendix C.
School Practice Documentation: Documenting and Organizing Quantitative Data

By Gloria Frolek Clark, Susan M. Cahill, and Carole Ivey

The occupational therapist uses information from many sources to gather quantitative and qualitative data about the curriculum, instruction, environment, and student.

Occupational therapists working in preschool or school environments gather data across multiple settings to facilitate participation and engagement within the student's educational environment (e.g., classroom, playground, cafeteria, bathroom, hallways). Documentation provides a critical chronological, legal record of occupational therapy services and student performance. One framework to organize and document these data efficiently is the Review, Interview, Observe, and Test (RIOT)/Instruction, Curriculum, Environment, Learner (ICEL) Matrix (Hosp, 2006, 2008; Wright, 2010). This framework allows the user to organize four potential sources of information (RIOT) within key domains of the education setting (ICEL). *Instruction* refers to how the content is taught, *curriculum* refers to what content is taught, *environment* refers to the context and conditions for learning, and *learner* refers to the student's unique capacities and traits. The learner is listed last on purpose; if the first three domains are "just right," the learner will learn.

The RIOT/ICEL matrix shares many of the same ideas as the *Occupational Therapy Practice Framework: Domain and Process, 3rd Edition* (American Occupational Therapy Association [AOTA], 2014a), including context/environments (environment); client factors, performance skills, and performance patterns (learner); and occupations and activities. Occupational therapists use data from these areas to determine the need for services as well as the effectiveness of services. (*Note:* Although occupational therapy assistants are actively involved in data collection and service delivery, for this article, the term *occupational therapist* is used because occupational therapists are responsible for all aspects of the service delivery process and must be directly involved during the initial evaluation and ongoing intervention as well as supervise the occupational therapy assistant [AOTA, 2014b]). Quantitative data should be gathered "for the purpose of establishing a baseline and monitoring the student's program" (Frolek Clark & Miller, 1996, p. 705).

When using the matrix, data may be entered in any order, but avoid leaving empty boxes. For example, an occupational therapist may begin with review and enter the information about the curriculum first, since he or she works in the district. Then the therapist may review the student's school educational record and enter pertinent data under instruction, environment, and learner. Each of these RIOT strategies will be further described. When data is applicable to more than one section, place it in only one. See Table 1 for examples.

Review

A complete and thorough record review provides information about the history and nature of the concern. Data, such as the number of days the student missed school, scores on state and previous assessments, office disciplinary referrals, report cards, portfolios, and medical and educational history, can be used in decision making. The purpose of reviewing these data is to determine supports or barriers to the student's current participation/performance and to gather baseline performance data.

Table 1. Sample of RIOT/ICEL Matrix Completed by an Occupational Therapist

Brad, Grade 1
All occupation areas were reviewed.
Ones that were problematic include: Social participation (sitting in seat) and Education (difficulty with fine motor/writing skills).

	Instruction	Curriculum	Environment	Learner
Review	Attended kindergarten last year	Handwriting Without Tears curriculum	28 students in this classroom	• No medical information in file • Education records indicate student missed 15 days of school
Interview	• Brad seems to learn better with teacher-directed and small-group format. • Teacher reports that following individual direction, Brad works for 3 minutes independently, then needs to be cued.	**School curriculum requires:** Write first name on the line, write lowercase letters within the lines, copy words from the board, write sentences in a journal. Complete fine motor activities (e.g., cutting out various pictures, coloring and drawing pictures, managing glue sticks).	Teacher reports large class size and increase in students (6) receiving special education services; very stressful without any other adults to help; feeling she can't help all of the kids.	**From Teacher:** • Brad typically stands by his desk to complete his work. • Brad frequently scribbles on his paper or tears it up. • Brad does well in academics, but has difficulty writing letters and numbers. • Brad is unable to write his first name on his paper; he frequently reverses lowercase letters. **From Parent:** • Brad refuses to do fine motor activities at home. He just wants to play on iPad.
Observe	Teacher frequently calls on students in the first row. Teacher asks a question and waits 5–7 seconds for a response.	Following class discussion, students were expected to complete a fill-in-the-blank worksheet using their sight word list.	• Brad sits near 3 other students who receive extra help for behavior and reading. They appear to be distractors for him working independently. • His seat is near the window, which appears to be a distractor. • Variety of writing materials and desk models available to support writing.	• Brad frequently needs 20–30 seconds to process auditory information before he is able to contribute to class discussions. • During 15 minutes, Brad completed only 1 of the 6 questions on worksheet (24:28 peers finished).

Test/Tools	Brad needs verbal instructions as well as modeling.	• **District writing probe during 1st quarter.** Brad wrote 6:26 lower case letters and 0:8 words. Peers scores ranged from 23 to 26 letters and 5 to 8 words.
		• **Portfolio review:** Brad did not write any legible sentences during 4 days of journaling, compared with 2 peers who each wrote 2 sentences; ranging from 4 to 6 words. Pictures were cut in half rather than following outline.
		• **Fine motor tasks—OT within the classroom (used classroom materials used within the classroom, led by OT):**
		  • *Cutting using classroom materials*—Brad cut off the animal's tail and had 8 errors that were 1/2" from the line (compared with 24:28 students' projects within 1/4" of the line).
		  • *Coloring using classroom materials*—Brad was outside of the picture borders for the entire picture (compared with 25:28 students who colored within at least 80% of the boundaries).
			When Brad sat in chair, he fell out 3 times when trying to color around edges. OT allowed Brad to choose sitting on an inflatable cushion, inflatable ball, or standing. He tried all 3 and sat on the inflatable ball. No falls occurred during the 4 minutes on the ball.	• Brad has difficulty using 2 sides of his body to complete tasks (e.g., hold paper and cut).
				• Easily frustrated with tasks that require dexterity and motor planning

Interview

Occupational therapists working in the schools are familiar with interviewing multiple sources when conducting student evaluations. However, the challenge in interviewing sources is gathering specific qualitative and quantitative data that will allow for identifying supports and barriers to occupational performance and for measuring progress (e.g., baseline and changes). Interview questions may be structured or informal and are typically open ended. Each source can contribute different information (e.g., parent, teacher, playground aide).

Current teachers, past teachers, teacher assistants, and the student will be able to provide information about the instruction, curriculum, environment, and typical routines during the school day. Whether the concern is academic or non-academic, knowing which skills are important to the teacher and the school is necessary (e.g., student should write his or her name, line up when the bell rings, put on a coat, change clothes after gym). Identifying the amount and type of instruction that has been provided allows the therapist to determine the effectiveness of the instruction. Learning about the structure, delivery, and routines of the instruction or program can help determine whether it was done with fidelity.

Qualitative data are often obtained during interviews and can be used to identify the strengths and needs within the ICEL domains. Using open-ended questions, such as, "Tell me about Stu's interactions with his peers and his friendships," provides information from various viewpoints. Because of personal bias and subjectivity to responses, it is important to cross reference the information gained through interviews with other sources, as well as the student's permanent records, and direct observation data. Quantitative data may also be obtained during the interview. For example, a teacher may refer to his or her grade book to identify the number of times a student has not handed in homework (compared with the class average).

To gather data on the learner, possible sources include teachers, teacher assistants, parents, past teachers, and the students themselves. Ask questions about educational, medical, and developmental history; motivation; and current academic and social behavior performance. After hearing qualitative data, such as, "Jesse has difficulty completing homework on time," probe deeper with questions to gather quantitative data, such as, "How many other students in your classroom are not turning in their homework?"

Observation

Occupational therapists play an integral role in collecting data as part of problem identification. Information gained from observations can lead to the educational team's better understanding of the cause of the student's academic, nonacademic, or behavioral problems. Observations can also assist the team in comparing the student's performance with that of his or her peers. "One of the important advantages of carefully executed quantitative observations is that the findings can serve as a baseline against which progress can be measured" (Coster & Frolek Clark, 2013, p. 90).

Structured observation should be planned carefully to identify the behavior in observable terms (putting on coat, sitting in chair, lining up, writing in journal) and within the typical context for observation. The type of measurement (e.g., time elapsed or frequency count) should be based on the type of performance. Direct observations should occur in the student's typical classroom environment within the natural routine, if possible. Use the four main components of ICEL to focus on the student's response to the teacher's instructional strategies, the student's ability to work through curricular exercises, the impact of the physical and social aspects of the environment on the student's learning and participation, and the student's unique characteristics (Wright, 2010).

The occupational therapist should approach direct observations systematically and select or devise quantitative methods that are appropriate for capturing the student's performance with certain tasks or in certain environments. Three examples of measurements by an occupational therapist may include

1. Interval recording data focusing on on-task behavior for a student with suspected attention problems by rating the student's behavior at specific intervals of time (e.g., every 3 minutes);
2. Duration data using the number of seconds (or minutes) a student with self-care difficulties needs to complete his or her morning routine (e.g., enter school building, go to locker, take off coat, hang up coat, take materials out of book bag, place book bag in locker, close locker door, enter classroom, sit in assigned seat); and
3. Frequency data focusing on recording/counting the frequency with which a student with suspected social and emotional difficulties initiates interactions with peers during recess.

All of these provide baseline as well as ongoing data for decision making.

Test

School-related performance tests and tools provide the team with information about the student's performance in schools. Occupational therapists may use the results from tests, classroom probes, or assessments normed for that district for evaluation, progress monitoring, or intervention planning. Occupational therapists should use tools designed to evaluate school-related performance (e.g., School Function Assessment; Coster, Deeney, Haltiwanger, & Haley, 1998). Our environment and context influence performance (AOTA, 2014a). Try various environmental adaptations, modifications, or equipment, and document changes in the student's performance.

Conclusion

The occupational therapist uses information from many sources (e.g., review, interview, observation, tests) to gather quantitative and qualitative data about the curriculum, instruction, environment, and the student. These data are used to make decisions about services, establish goals, monitor the student's progress on meeting these goals, and determine effectiveness of occupational therapy intervention.

References

American Occupational Therapy Association. (2014a). Occupational therapy practice framework: Domain and process (3rd ed.). *American Journal of Occupational Therapy, 50,* S1–S48. http://dx.doi.org/10.5014/ajot.2014.682006

American Occupational Therapy Association. (2014b). Guidelines for supervision, roles, and responsibilities during the delivery of occupational therapy services. *American Journal of Occupational Therapy, 68,* S16–22. http://dx.doi.org/10.5014/ajot.2014.686S03

Coster, W., Deeney, T., Haltiwanger, J., & Haley, S. (1998). *School Function Assessment.* San Antonio, TX: Psychological Corporation.

Coster, W., & Frolek Clark, G. (2013). Best Practices in school occupational therapy evaluation to support participation. In G. Frolek Clark & B. Chandler (Eds.), *Best practices for occupational therapy in schools* (pp. 83–93). Bethesda, MD: AOTA Press.

Frolek Clark, G., & Miller, L. (1996). Providing effective occupational therapy services: Data-based decision making in school-based practice. *American Journal of Occupational Therapy, 50,* 701–708.

Hosp, J. L. (2006) Implementing RTI: Assessment practices and response to intervention. *NASP Communiqué, 34*(7). Retrieved from http://www.nasponline.org/publications/cq/cq347rti.aspx

Hosp, J. L. (2008). Best practices in aligning academic assessment with instruction. In A. Thomas & J. Grimes (Eds.), *Best practices in school psychology V* (pp. 363–376). Bethesda, MD: National Association of School Psychologists.

Wright, J. (2010). *The RIOT/ICEL Matrix: Organizing data to answer questions about student academic performance & behavior.* Retrieved from http://www.interventioncentral.org/sites/default/files/rti_riot_icel_data_collection.pdf

Appendix D.
Guidelines for Supervision, Roles, and Responsibilities During the Delivery of Occupational Therapy Services

This document is a set of guidelines describing the supervision, roles, and responsibilities of occupational therapy practitioners. Intended for both internal and external audiences, it also provides an outline of the roles and responsibilities of occupational therapists, occupational therapy assistants, and occupational therapy aides during the delivery of occupational therapy services.

General Supervision

These guidelines provide a definition of supervision and outline parameters regarding effective supervision as it relates to the delivery of occupational therapy services. The guidelines themselves cannot be interpreted to constitute a standard of supervision in any particular locality. Occupational therapists, occupational therapy assistants, and occupational therapy aides are expected to meet applicable state and federal regulations, adhere to relevant workplace and payer policies and to the *Occupational Therapy Code of Ethics and Ethics Standards* (American Occupational Therapy Association [AOTA], 2010), and participate in ongoing professional development activities to maintain continuing competency.

Within the scope of occupational therapy practice, *supervision* is a process aimed at ensuring the safe and effective delivery of occupational therapy services and fostering professional competence and development. In addition, in these guidelines, supervision is viewed as a cooperative process in which two or more people participate in a joint effort to establish, maintain, and/or elevate a level of competence and performance. Supervision is based on mutual understanding between the supervisor and the supervisee about each other's competence, experience, education, and credentials. It fosters growth and development, promotes effective utilization of resources, encourages creativity and innovation, and provides education and support to achieve a goal.

Supervision of Occupational Therapists and Occupational Therapy Assistants

Occupational Therapists

Based on education and training, occupational therapists, after initial certification and relevant state licensure or other governmental requirements, are autonomous practitioners who are able to deliver occupational therapy services independently. Occupational therapists are responsible for all aspects of occupational therapy service delivery and are accountable for the safety and effectiveness of occupational therapy services and the service delivery process. Occupational therapists are encouraged to seek peer supervision and mentoring for ongoing development of best practice approaches and to promote professional growth.

Occupational Therapy Assistants

Based on education and training, occupational therapy assistants, after initial certification and meeting of state regulatory requirements, must receive supervision from an occupational therapist to deliver occupational therapy services. Occupational therapy assistants deliver occupational therapy services under the supervision of and in partnership with occupational therapists. Occupational therapists and occupational therapy assistants are equally responsible for developing a collaborative plan for supervision. The occupational therapist is ultimately responsible for the implementation of appropriate supervision, but the occupational therapy assistant also has a responsibility to seek and obtain appropriate supervision to ensure proper occupational therapy is being provided.

General Principles

1. Supervision involves guidance and oversight related to the delivery of occupational therapy services and the facilitation of professional growth and competence. It is the responsibility of the occupational therapy assistant to seek the appropriate quality and frequency of supervision to ensure safe and effective occupational therapy service delivery. It is the responsibility of the occupational therapist to provide adequate and appropriate supervision.

2. To ensure safe and effective occupational therapy services, it is the responsibility of occupational therapists to recognize when they require peer supervision or mentoring that supports current and advancing levels of competence and professional growth.

3. The specific frequency, methods, and content of supervision may vary and are dependent on the

    a. Complexity of client needs,

    b. Number and diversity of clients,

    c. Knowledge and skill level of the occupational therapist and the occupational therapy assistant,

    d. Type of practice setting,

    e. Requirements of the practice setting, and

    f. Other regulatory requirements.

4. Supervision of the occupational therapy assistant that is more frequent than the minimum level required by the practice setting or regulatory requirements may be necessary when

    a. The needs of the client and the occupational therapy process are complex and changing,

    b. The practice setting provides occupational therapy services to a large number of clients with diverse needs, or

    c. The occupational therapist and occupational therapy assistant determine that additional supervision is necessary to ensure safe and effective delivery of occupational therapy services.

5. There are a variety of types and methods of supervision. Methods can include but are not limited to direct, face-to-face contact and indirect contact. Examples of methods or types of supervision that involve direct face-to-face contact include observation, modeling, client demonstration, discussions, teaching, and instruction. Examples of methods or types of supervision that involve indirect contact include phone conversations, written correspondence, and electronic exchanges.

6. Occupational therapists and occupational therapy assistants must abide by facility and state requirements regarding the documentation of a supervision plan and supervision contacts. Documentation may include the

    a. Frequency of supervisory contact,

    b. Methods or types of supervision,

    c. Content areas addressed,

    d. Evidence to support areas and levels of competency, and

    e. Names and credentials of the persons participating in the supervisory process.

7. Peer supervision and mentoring related to professional growth, such as leadership and advocacy skills development, may differ from the peer supervision mentoring needed to provide occupational therapy services. The person

providing this supervision, as well as the frequency, method, and content of supervision, should be responsive to the supervisee's advancing levels of professional growth.

Supervision Outside the Delivery of Occupational Therapy Services

The education and expertise of occupational therapists and occupational therapy assistants prepare them for employment in arenas other than those related to the delivery of occupational therapy. In these other arenas, supervision may be provided by non–occupational therapy professionals.

1. The guidelines of the setting, regulatory agencies, and funding agencies direct the supervision requirements.

2. The occupational therapist and occupational therapy assistant should obtain and use credentials or job titles commensurate with their roles in these other employment arenas.

3. The following can be used to determine whether the services provided are related to the delivery of occupational therapy:

    a. State practice acts;

    b. Regulatory agency standards and rules;

    c. *Occupational Therapy Practice Framework: Domain and Process* (AOTA, 2014) and other AOTA official documents; and

    d. Written and verbal agreement among the occupational therapist, the occupational therapy assistant, the client, and the agency or payer about the services provided.

Roles and Responsibilities of Occupational Therapists and Occupational Therapy Assistants During the Delivery of Occupational Therapy Services

Overview

The focus of occupational therapy is to assist the client in "achieving health, well-being, and participation in life through engagement in occupation" (AOTA, 2014, p. S2). Occupational therapy addresses the needs and goals of the client related to engaging in areas of occupation and considers the performance skills, performance patterns, context and environment, and client factors that may influence performance in various areas of occupation.

1. The occupational therapist is responsible for all aspects of occupational therapy service delivery and is accountable for the safety and effectiveness of the occupational therapy service delivery process. The occupational therapy service delivery process involves evaluation, intervention planning, intervention implementation, intervention review, and targeting of outcomes and outcomes evaluation.

2. The occupational therapist must be directly involved in the delivery of services during the initial evaluation and regularly throughout the course of intervention, intervention review, and outcomes evaluation.

3. The occupational therapy assistant delivers safe and effective occupational therapy services under the supervision of and in partnership with the occupational therapist.

4. It is the responsibility of the occupational therapist to determine when to delegate responsibilities to an occupational therapy assistant. It is the responsibility of the occupational therapy assistant who performs the delegated responsibilities to demonstrate service competency and also to not accept delegated responsibilities that go beyond the scope of an occupational therapy assistant.

5. The occupational therapist and the occupational therapy assistant demonstrate and document service competency for clinical reasoning and judgment during the service delivery process as well as for the performance of specific techniques, assessments, and intervention methods used.

6. When delegating aspects of occupational therapy services, the occupational therapist considers the following factors:

   a. Complexity of the client's condition and needs,

   b. Knowledge, skill, and competence of the occupational therapy assistant,

   c. Nature and complexity of the intervention,

   d. Needs and requirements of the practice setting, and

   e. Appropriate scope of practice of an occupational therapy assistant under state law and other requirements.

Roles and Responsibilities

Regardless of the setting in which occupational therapy services are delivered, occupational therapists and occupational therapy assistants assume the following general responsibilities during evaluation; intervention planning, implementation, and review; and targeting and evaluating outcomes.

Evaluation

1. The occupational therapist directs the evaluation process.

2. The occupational therapist is responsible for directing all aspects of the initial contact during the occupational therapy evaluation, including

   a. Determining the need for service,

   b. Defining the problems within the domain of occupational therapy to be addressed,

   c. Determining the client's goals and priorities,

   d. Establishing intervention priorities,

   e. Determining specific further assessment needs, and

   f. Determining specific assessment tasks that can be delegated to the occupational therapy assistant.

3. The occupational therapist initiates and directs the evaluation, interprets the data, and develops the intervention plan.

4. The occupational therapy assistant contributes to the evaluation process by implementing delegated assessments and by providing verbal and written reports of observations, assessments, and client capacities to the occupational therapist.

5. The occupational therapist interprets the information provided by the occupational therapy assistant and integrates that information into the evaluation and decision-making process.

Intervention Planning

1. The occupational therapist has overall responsibility for the development of the occupational therapy intervention plan.

2. The occupational therapist and the occupational therapy assistant collaborate with the client to develop the plan.

3. The occupational therapy assistant is responsible for being knowledgeable about evaluation results and for providing input into the intervention plan, based on client needs and priorities.

Intervention Implementation

1. The occupational therapist has overall responsibility for intervention implementation.

2. When delegating aspects of the occupational therapy intervention to the occupational therapy assistant, the occupational therapist is responsible for providing appropriate supervision.

3. The occupational therapy assistant is responsible for being knowledgeable about the client's occupational therapy goals.

4. The occupational therapy assistant in collaboration with the occupational therapist selects, implements, and makes modifications to occupational therapy interventions, including, but not limited to, occupations and activities, preparatory methods and tasks, client education and training, and group interventions consistent with demonstrated competency levels, client goals, and the requirements of the practice setting.

Intervention Review

1. The occupational therapist is responsible for determining the need for continuing, modifying, or discontinuing occupational therapy services.

2. The occupational therapy assistant contributes to this process by exchanging information with and providing documentation to the occupational therapist about the client's responses to and communications during intervention.

Targeting and Evaluating Outcomes

1. The occupational therapist is responsible for selecting, measuring, and interpreting outcomes that are related to the client's ability to engage in occupations.

2. The occupational therapy assistant is responsible for being knowledgeable about the client's targeted occupational therapy outcomes and for providing information and documentation related to outcome achievement.

3. The occupational therapy assistant may implement outcome measurements and provide needed client discharge resources.

Supervision of Occupational Therapy Aides[1]

An *aide,* as used in occupational therapy practice, is an individual who provides supportive services to the occupational therapist and the occupational therapy assistant. Aides do not provide skilled occupational therapy services. An aide is trained by an occupational therapist or an occupational therapy assistant to perform specifically delegated tasks. The occupational therapist is responsible for the overall use and actions of the aide. An aide first must demonstrate competency to be able to perform the assigned, delegated client and non-client tasks.

1. The occupational therapist must oversee the development, documentation, and implementation of a plan to supervise and routinely assess the ability of the occupational therapy aide to carry out non–client- and client-related tasks. The occupational therapy assistant may contribute to the development and documentation of this plan.

2. The occupational therapy assistant can supervise the aide.

3. *Non–client-related tasks* include clerical and maintenance activities and preparation of the work area or equipment.

4. *Client-related tasks* are routine tasks during which the aide may interact with the client. The following factors must be present when an occupational therapist or occupational therapy assistant delegates a selected client-related task to the aide:

   a. The outcome anticipated for the delegated task is predictable.

   b. The situation of the client and the environment is stable and will not require that judgment, interpretations, or adaptations be made by the aide.

   c. The client has demonstrated some previous performance ability in executing the task.

   d. The task routine and process have been clearly established.

---

[1]Depending on the setting in which service is provided, aides may be referred to by various names. Examples include, but are not limited to, *rehabilitation aides, restorative aides, extenders, paraprofessionals,* and *rehab techs* (AOTA, 2009).

5. When performing delegated client-related tasks, the supervisor must ensure that the aide

   a. Is trained and able to demonstrate competency in carrying out the selected task and using equipment, if appropriate;

   b. Has been instructed on how to specifically carry out the delegated task with the specific client; and

   c. Knows the precautions, signs, and symptoms for the particular client that would indicate the need to seek assistance from the occupational therapist or occupational therapy assistant.

6. The supervision of the aide needs to be documented. Documentation includes information about frequency and methods of supervision used, the content of supervision, and the names and credentials of all persons participating in the supervisory process.

Summary

These guidelines about supervision, roles, and responsibilities are to assist in the appropriate utilization of occupational therapists, occupational therapy assistants, and occupational therapy aides and in the appropriate and effective provision of occupational therapy services. It is expected that occupational therapy services are delivered in accordance with applicable state and federal regulations, relevant workplace policies, the *Occupational Therapy Code of Ethics and Ethics Standards* (AOTA, 2010), and continuing competency and professional development guidelines. For information regarding the supervision of occupational therapy students, please refer to *Fieldwork Level II and Occupational Therapy Students: A Position Paper* (AOTA, 2012).

References

American Occupational Therapy Association. (2009). Guidelines for supervision, roles, and responsibilities during the delivery of occupational therapy services. *American Journal of Occupational Therapy, 63,* 797–803. http://dx.doi.org/10/5014/ajot.63.6.797

American Occupational Therapy Association. (2010). Occupational therapy code of ethics and ethics standards (2010). *American Journal of Occupational Therapy, 64*(6, Suppl.), S17–S26. http://dx.doi.org/10.5014/ajot.2010.64S17

American Occupational Therapy Association. (2012). Fieldwork Level II and occupational therapy students: A position paper. *American Journal of Occupational Therapy, 66*(6, Suppl.), S75–S77. http://dx.doi.org/10.5014/ajot.2012.66S75

American Occupational Therapy Association. (2014). Occupational therapy practice framework: Domain and process (3rd ed.). *American Journal of Occupational Therapy, 68*(Suppl. 1), S1–S48. http://dx.doi.org/10.5014/ajot.2014.682005

Additional Reading

American Occupational Therapy Association. (2010). Standards of practice for occupational therapy. *American Journal of Occupational Therapy, 64*(Suppl.), S106–S111. http://dx.doi.org/10.5014/ajot.2010.64S106

Authors
Sara Jane Brayman, PhD, OTR/L, FAOTA
Gloria Frolek Clark, MS, OTR/L, FAOTA
Janet V. DeLany, DEd, OTR/L
Eileen R. Garza, PhD, OTR, ATP
Mary V. Radomski, MA, OTR/L, FAOTA
Ruth Ramsey, MS, OTR/L
Carol Siebert, MS, OTR/L
Kristi Voelkerding, BS, COTA/L
Patricia D. LaVesser, PhD, OTR/L, *SIS Liaison*
Lenna Aird, *ASD Liaison*
Deborah Lieberman, MHSA, OTR/L, FAOTA, *AOTA Headquarters Liaison*

for

The Commission on Practice
Sara Jane Brayman, PhD, OTR/L, FAOTA, *Chairperson*

Adopted by the Representative Assembly 2004C24

Edited by the Commission on Practice 2014
Debbie Amini, EdD, OTR/L, CHT, FAOTA, *Chairperson*

Adopted by the Representative Assembly Coordinating Council (RACC) for the Representative Assembly, 2014.

Citation. American Occupational Therapy Association. (2014). Guidelines for supervision, roles, and responsibilities during the delivery of occupational therapy services. *American Journal of Occupational Therapy, 68*(Suppl. 3), S16–S22. https://doi.org/10.5014/ajot.2014.686S03

Appendix E.
AOTA Resources for School-Based Practice and Documentation

The American Occupational Therapy Association (AOTA) has resources for members and nonmembers.

AOTA Professional Documents

AOTA official documents are on 5-year review cycles. They are available to members in the *American Journal of Occupational Therapy* at http://08journal.net

AOTA Website (www.aota.org)

AOTA members and nonmembers can find various articles, tip sheets, fact sheets, and other information at these websites:

- **Children and Youth:** Includes resources related to autism, caseload to workload, distinct value, literacy, school-based practice, and so on—http://www.aota.org/Practice/Children-Youth.aspx

- **Mental Health:** Includes evidence-based practice information and resources on mental health, such as access to articles, tip sheets, fact sheets, and apps—http://www.aota.org/Practice/Mental-Health.aspx

- **Evidence-Based Practice and Research:** Provides information on various topics, a researcher database, evidence exchange, research opportunities, and resource directory—http://www.aota.org/Practice/Researchers.aspx

- **Publications and News:** Includes the *American Journal of Occupational Therapy, OT Practice* magazine, *SIS Quarterly* newsletters, and e-newsletters—http://www.aota.org/Publications-News.aspx

- **Information about occupational therapy for professionals:** In addition to information about occupational therapy, the left column offers links to information for professionals about various topics such as those above, health and wellness, and ethics—http://www.aota.org/About-Occupational-Therapy/Professionals.aspx

- **Information about occupational therapy for patients and clients:** Provides a caregiver toolkit and various resources in the Children and Youth section that are relevant for teachers and families, including the childhood occupations toolkit, tips about autism, and tips for children in school—http://www.aota.org/About-Occupational-Therapy/Patients-Clients.aspx

Books and Continuing Education

- Frolek Clark, G., & Chandler, B. (Eds.). (2013). *Best practices for occupational therapy in schools,* Bethesda, MD: AOTA Press.

  - This book offers many chapters on evaluation, response to intervention, documentation, and so on. Each chapter is also available as continuing education from AOTA Learn.

- Hanft, B., & Shepherd, B. (Eds.) (2016). *Collaborating for student success* (2nd ed.). Bethesda, MD: AOTA Press.
  - Provides practical, real-world guidance on how to collaborate with students, families, and school personnel to support student performance, participation, and success.
- Jackson, L. (2007). *Occupational therapy services for children and youth under IDEA* (3rd ed.). Bethesda, MD: AOTA Press.
  - Provides information and resources about IDEA and occupational therapy practice in schools, preschools, early intervention, and other settings such as child care.

These books and continuing education opportunities can be found at store.aota.org.

Social Media

OT Connections is a social media platform that can be used to share questions or information about all areas of practice, including documentation and forms. There are public groups and forums available to nonmembers and member forums that are offered as a member benefit. Visit https://otconnections.aota.org

Appendix F.
AOTA Occupational Profile Template

AOTA OCCUPATIONAL PROFILE TEMPLATE

"The occupational profile is a summary of a client's occupational history and experiences, patterns of daily living, interests, values, and needs" (AOTA, 2014, p. S13). The information is obtained from the client's perspective through both formal interview techniques and casual conversation and leads to an individualized, client-centered approach to intervention.

Each item below should be addressed to complete the occupational profile. Page numbers are provided to reference a description in the *Occupational Therapy Practice Framework: Domain and Process, 3rd Edition* (AOTA, 2014).

Client Report	**Reason the client is seeking service and concerns related to engagement in occupations**	Why is the client seeking service, and what are the client's current concerns relative to engaging in occupations and in daily life activities? (This may include the client's general health status.)
	Occupations in which the client is successful (p. S5)	In what occupations does the client feel successful, and what barriers are affecting his or her success?
	Personal interests and values (p. S7)	What are the client's values and interests?
	Occupational history (i.e., life experiences)	What is the client's occupational history (i.e., life experiences)?
	Performance patterns (routines, roles, habits, & rituals) (p. S8)	What are the client's patterns of engagement in occupations, and how have they changed over time? What are the client's daily life roles? (Patterns can support or hinder occupational performance.)

		What aspects of the client's environments or contexts does he or she see as:	
		Supports to Occupational Engagement	**Barriers to Occupational Engagement**
Environment	**Physical (p. S28) (e.g., buildings, furniture, pets)**		
	Social (p. S28) (e.g., spouse, friends, caregivers)		
Context	**Cultural (p. S28) (e.g., customs, beliefs)**		
	Personal (p. S28) (e.g., age, gender, SES, education)		
	Temporal (p. S28) (e.g., stage of life, time, year)		
	Virtual (p. S28) (e.g., chat, email, remote monitoring)		
Client Goals	**Client's priorities and desired targeted outcomes: (p. S34)**	Consider: occupational performance—improvement and enhancement, prevention, participation, role competence, health and wellness, quality of life, well-being, and/or occupational justice.	

ADDITIONAL RESOURCES

For a complete description of each component and examples of each, refer to the *Occupational Therapy Practice Framework: Domain and Process, 3rd Edition.*

American Occupational Therapy Association. (2014). Occupational therapy practice framework: Domain and process (3rd ed.). *American Journal of Occupational Therapy, 68*, S1–S48. https://doi.org/10.5014/ajot.2014.682006

The occupational profile is a requirement of the *CPT®* occupational therapy evaluation codes as of January 1, 2017. For more information visit www.aota.org/coding.

Appendix G.
New Occupational Therapy Evaluation Coding Overview

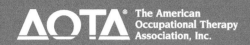

New Occupational Therapy Evaluation Coding Overview

On January 1, 2017, new codes will go into effect for occupational therapy evaluations. The American Medical Association (AMA) *Common Procedural Terminology (CPT®)* 2017 manual will list three levels of occupational therapy evaluation and one level of re-evaluation under the Physical Medicine and Rehabilitation (PM&R) section of the manual (or codebook). The previous codes have been redefined and assigned new numbers with new requirements.

To use the correct code in the new system, occupational therapists will have to attend to new criteria that distinguish differing levels of evaluation. This document is intended to provide an overview of the codes to assist occupational therapists with making correct coding choices that reflect modern occupational therapy practice. The new CPT® codes describe differences in complexity of evaluations, ranging from low (i.e., straightforward), to moderate (i.e., involved), to high (i.e., very complex). Previously, when an occupational therapist performed an evaluation of a client, only one code (97003) was available to reflect the clinical work accomplished during that evaluation session.

The new evaluation codes (97165, 97166, and 97167) will replace CPT® code 97003 and offer three levels of an occupational therapy evaluation: low, moderate, and high. There is one re-evaluation code (97168).

The code descriptors as published in the CPT® manual are available on AOTA's website at www.aota.org. New manuals are available in print and online from the AMA.

The new codes were developed through a process involving the AMA (which develops, publishes, and owns the CPT® system), the American Occupational Therapy Association (AOTA), and other professional societies. Payers, including Medicare, Medicaid, and insurance providers, use these codes to identify services for payment.

Medicare will begin using these codes on January 1, 2017, and most other third-party payers (e.g., Medicaid, insurers) will follow this procedure by developing individual payer policies on use of and payment for codes.

HOW CPT® DESCRIBES THE OCCUPATIONAL THERAPY EVALUATION AND REEVALUTION CODES

First, it is important to review and understand the precise language in the 2017 AMA CPT® manual. It provides the following introduction to the codes for Occupational Therapy Evaluation:

> *Occupational therapy evaluations include an occupational profile, medical and therapy history, relevant assessments, and development of a plan of care, which reflects the therapist's clinical reasoning and interpretation of the data. Coordination, consideration, and collaboration of care with physicians, other qualified health care professionals, or agencies is provided consistent with the nature of the problem(s) and the needs of the patient, family, and/or other caregivers. (p. 664)*

The definition follows the approach to evaluation in the Occupational Therapy Practice Framework: Domain and Process (3rd ed.; AOTA, 2014). The Framework will be referenced throughout this document, as it provides important direction for conducting appropriate, best-practice evaluations.

The new descriptions in CPT® set the stage for promoting optimal occupational therapy practice. By conducting a profile, doing standardized and other tests and measures, and showing the breadth of concerns occupational therapy considers, we promote distinct value. The evaluation process can communicate to others the full scope of occupational therapy practice. The codes can be a tool to promote distinct value.

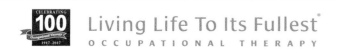

4720 Montgomery Lane, Bethesda, MD 20814-3425
Phone: 301-652-2682 TDD: 800-377-8555 Fax: 301-652-7711

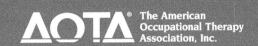

DETERMINING THE CORRECT LEVEL OF EVALUATION

The Code Language on Levels

In these new codes, the CPT® describes exactly what should be done in an evaluation:

- Occupational profile and client history (medical and therapy)
- Assessments of occupational performance
- Clinical decision making
- Development of plan of care

Identifying and Reporting the complexity level of an evaluation focuses on the first three of these factor—profile and history, assessment and determination of deficits, and clinical decision making. These three factors must be "scored" and defensible documentation written to support the choice of a level. The development of the Plan of Care (POC) is part of the overall evaluation process and must reflect how and why you scored the evaluation as high, moderate or low.

The three components are the factors that payers and others will review to assure the therapist has chosen the right code level. But in a best practice occupational therapy evaluation, all the factors are integrated. In best practice, for instance, clinical decision making transcends all parts of the evaluation. How assessments are conducted is related to the determination of performance limitations and deficits. Best occupational therapy practice recognizes that all three CPT® factors that determine a level are integrated into a holistic evaluation, and that other factors, such as age or environment, are also considered. The plan of care reflects the process and outcomes of the therapist's attention to each of the CPT® factors in the context of the whole evaluation to meet the patient's or client's needs.

The CPT® requirements do not mean that a therapist provides an evaluation using only these three components. The three components are what must be validated in choosing a level but a sufficient evaluation must be provided as appropriate to occupational therapy practice. Why a particular level was chosen should be supported in the documentation of the evaluation.

The codes direct that each component must be given a level. The level is most likely determined after completion of the evaluation, but therapists should be familiar with the criteria at the start so they can be considering the level as they proceed through the evaluation.

Choose a Level That is Appropriate

Levels must be determined specifically for each of the three components in order to choose the correct code. In order to move to a higher level of evaluation all three components must be of the higher level. For example, if the profile and history are moderate and the assessment and identification of deficits in occupational performance is moderate, but the clinical decision making component is high, the evaluation must still be coded moderate. Therapists must

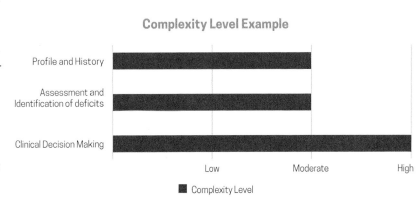

Complexity Level Example

	Low	Moderate	High
Profile and History			
Assessment and Identification of deficits			
Clinical Decision Making			

■ Complexity Level

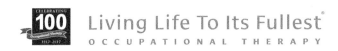

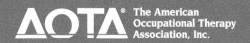

remember that they are ethically, and in some cases legally, required to choose and report the correct code. The code design considers the presenting patient condition, the analytical work of the therapist, and assessment and identification of the scope and nature of the client's/patient's performance concerns and goals. A proper evaluation involves a broader view and other components. But choosing a level is necessary to report the correct code.

Each of the three components that affect the code level is discussed below *following the language of the actual code descriptors in the manual.*

1. Profile and History

Was an occupational profile completed? How complex is the client history (medical and therapy) to meet the client needs?

The occupational therapy process as described in the Framework is reflected in the code language, especially in its requirement of completing an occupational profile as well as a medical and therapy history. The therapist uses the occupational profile to frame the evaluation around the client. Determining the level considers how involved both the profile and history must be to determine the code level. The code descriptor categorizes this component by whether these two elements are problem focused, detailed, or comprehensive. This table provides the language from the AMA CPT® manual describing the levels of profile and history.

CPT® Code	CPT® Descriptors
Low Complexity (97165)	An occupational profile and medical and therapy history, which includes a **brief** history including review of medical and/or therapy records relating to the presenting problem.
Moderate Complexity (97166)	An occupational profile and medical and therapy history, which includes an **expanded** review of medical and/or therapy records and additional review of physical, cognitive, or psychosocial history related to current functional performance.
High Complexity (97167)	An occupational profile and medical and therapy history, which includes review of medical and/or therapy records and **extensive** additional review of physical, cognitive, or psychosocial history related to current functional performance.

The key words in CPT® to consider when differentiating and choosing a level for this component are:

- Brief (Low)
- Expanded (Moderate)
- Extensive (High)

Occupational Profile

The occupational profile provides an understanding of the client's occupational history and experiences, patterns of daily living, interests, values, and needs. The client's problems and concerns about performing occupations and daily life activities are identified. The client's priorities for outcomes are determined.

To determine the level of occupational profile that must be completed, the therapist must consider the presenting problem(s), the reason(s) for referral, and the client's goals. Although a client may have multiple diagnoses, and be very complex, if he or she is in a stable state and wants one small or targeted issue addressed by the occupational therapy intervention, then this component should be coded as low complexity.

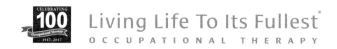

Living Life To Its Fullest®
OCCUPATIONAL THERAPY

4720 Montgomery Lane, Bethesda, MD 20814-3425
Phone: 301-652-2682 TDD: 800-377-8555 Fax: 301-652-7711

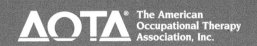

Client Medical History

The *client's history*, both medical and therapy, is reviewed and considered to identify aspects such as the prior level of function and presenting diagnosis that is causing the client to seek occupational therapy services. How much of the history is necessary depends on what the client is seeking services for and what the occupational therapist needs to know to continue with assessment and development of the plan of care. The referral for therapy may also provide additional information. It can also come from medical records of past and current care.

2. Assessment of Occupational Performance

How is the assessment of activity/participation restrictions described? How are performance deficits defined? How are performance deficits identified and counted?

The second criterion that must be considered in determining the level of the evaluation considers factors related to both the assessment process and the identification of what the code language calls performance deficits. Performance deficits are defined as activity limitations and/or participation restrictions that result from skills deficits. In the code language, these should be interpreted as occupations in which the client is experiencing problems. Occupations are defined in the *Occupational Therapy Practice Framework, Table 1*. This linkage between performance and skills deficits supports the emphasis of occupational therapy on occupational performance.

The code language specifies how to rate low, moderate and high evaluations in relation to assessments and identification of performance deficits—occupational areas in which there are deficits. Following is the actual code descriptor language:

CPT° Code	CPT° Descriptors
Low Complexity (97165)	An assessment(s) that identifies **1–3 performance deficits** (i.e., relating to physical cognitive or psychosocial skills) that result in activity limitations and/or participation restrictions
Moderate Complexity (97166)	An assessment(s) that identifies **3–5 performance deficits** (i.e., relating to physical cognitive or psychosocial skills) that result in activity limitations and/or participation restrictions
High Complexity (97167)	An assessment(s) that identifies **5 or more performance deficits** (i.e., relating to physical cognitive or psychosocial skills) that result in activity limitations and/or participation restrictions

Identification, Assessment, and Determination

The therapist should consider all the information gathered in the history and occupational profile and the data from the assessment process, to determine (with the client) the priority of occupational performance deficits to be addressed. Factors, such as client capacity and endurance, as well as any specification of deficits or restrictions in the referral, will influence how many performance deficits (occupations) will be addressed in the episode **for which this evaluation is being done.**

Ideally, the therapist will use standardized assessments to identify a performance deficit (activity limitation and/or participation restriction in occupations), and then decide with the client if that deficit is to be addressed. Performance deficits may also be identified by other assessment processes, although many payers are beginning to require standardized approaches. In addition, the evaluation must clearly document the identification and assessment of client factors, performance patterns as well as context and environment as they impact activity and participation. The Framework's Tables 2, 3, 4, and 5 are references for these terms.

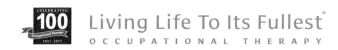

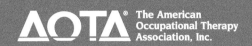

AOTA® The American
Occupational Therapy
Association, Inc.

www.aota.org

New Occupational Therapy Evaluation Coding Overview

How Does CPT® Describe Levels of Assessment?

The CPT® language for clinical decision making, discussed later, includes language that can be applied to thinking about how targeted or extensive assessments are. This language emphasizes the importance of both the collection of data and its analysis. The Table below provides language from the clinical decision making section that is pertinent to conducting the assessments.

CPT® Code	CPT® Descriptors
Low Complexity (97165)	Analysis of data from **problem-focused** assessment(s)
Moderate Complexity (97166)	Analysis of data from **detailed** assessment(s)
High Complexity (97167)	Analysis of data from **comprehensive** assessment(s)

The key words to consider from CPT® in differentiating levels concepts regarding the analysis are:

- Problem focused

- Detailed

- Comprehensive

What are Performance Deficits?

To emphasize: "performance deficits" in the code language should be interpreted as occupations in which the client is experiencing problems as defined in the *Occupational Therapy Practice Framework*, Table 1. The CPT® introduction to the codes identifies and defines skill areas including physical, cognitive, and psychosocial skills (see below) that affect performance of occupations. Performance deficits should be interpreted to be occupations, as they are defined in the Framework Table 1, in which there are activity limitations and/or participation restrictions. Performance deficits in occupations can be identified from this list as well as from the client's desired goals. Defining deficits in the CPT® **context is viewed as the process of identifying what areas of occupation or occupational therapy goals the plan of care will address.**

CPT® Definition of Performance Deficits	Introduction: Performance deficits refer to the inability to complete activities due to the lack of skills in one or more of the categories below (i.e. relating to physical, cognitive, or psychosocial skills).
AOTA Framework Definition of Occupations	OCCUPATIONS are various kinds of life activities in which individuals, groups, or populations engage, including activities of daily living, instrumental activities of daily living, rest and sleep, education, work, play, leisure, and social participation.

The code descriptor also provides definitions of areas in which the client may have limitations or performance in a broad way, supporting the full scope of occupational therapy.

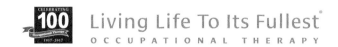

100 CELEBRATING 1917-2017   **Living Life To Its Fullest®**
OCCUPATIONAL THERAPY

4720 Montgomery Lane, Bethesda, MD 20814-3425
Phone: 301-652-2682 TDD: 800-377-8555 Fax: 301-652-7711

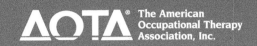

CPT° Skill Areas	CPT° Descriptors of Skill Areas
Physical	*Physical skills refer to impairments of* body structure or body function (e.g., balance, mobility, strength, endurance, fine or gross motor coordination, sensation, dexterity).* * AOTA regards "impairments of" as a typographical error and will be seeking revision because skills are not impairments.
Cognitive	Cognitive skills refer to the ability to attend, perceive, think, understand, problem solve, mentally sequence, learn, and remember, resulting in the ability to organize occupational performance in a timely and safe manner. These skills are observed when a person (1) attends to and selects, interacts with, and uses task tools and materials; (2) carries out individual actions and steps; and (3) modifies performance when problems are encountered.
Psychosocial	Psychosocial skills refer to interpersonal interactions, habits, routines and behaviors, active use of coping strategies, and/or environmental adaptations to develop skills necessary to successfully and appropriately participate in everyday tasks and social situations.

Again, the Framework is a reference. The terms in the CPT® relate to the Performance Skills described in Table 3 of the Framework.

AOTA Performance Skill Areas	AOTA Descriptors of Performance Skill Areas
Motor	**Motor Skills**— "Occupational performance skills observed as the person interacts with and moves task objects and self around the task environment" (e.g. activity of daily living [ADL] motor skills, school motor skills: Boyt, Gillen & Scaffa, 2014a, p.1237).
Process	**Process Skills**— "Occupational performance skills [e.g. ADL process skills, school process skills] observed as the person (1) selects, interacts with, and uses task tools and materials; (2) carries out individual actions and steps; and (3) modifies performance when problems are encountered" (Boyt Schell et al.,2014a, p. 1239).
Social Interaction	**Social Interaction Skills**— "Occupational performance skills observed during the ongoing stream of asocial exchange" (Boyt Schell et al., 2014a, p. 1241).

In addition, the evaluation must clearly document the identification and assessment of client factors, performance patterns, as well as context and environment as they impact activity and participation. The Framework's Tables 2,3, and 5 are references for these terms.

It is important to understand that the count of performance deficits or occupations in which the client is having difficulty is only one factor in assigning the level of the code. This is not the sole factor to determining the overall level. The complexity of the occupational profile and medical history, and the complexity of the clinical reasoning, which result in the development of the plan of care, must also be considered.

The number of deficits is, however, very important and will likely receive scrutiny as these new codes are used. Clinical judgment about the overall needs of the client, the expectations for this episode of care, and the overall complexity of the presenting client situation will dictate the number identified. This allows the therapist to use reasoning and judgment to identify the occupations impacted

The Framework and occupational therapy practice focus on the capacities of clients and their skills or potential skills related to occupational performance. Using occupational areas as what is counted retains the focus of the evaluation and treatment on occupation.

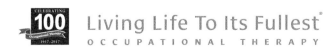

Living Life To Its Fullest®
OCCUPATIONAL THERAPY

4720 Montgomery Lane, Bethesda, MD 20814-3425
Phone: 301-652-2682 TDD: 800-377-8555 Fax: 301-652-7711

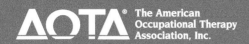

3. Level of Clinical Decision Making

What skills must the therapist use? How difficult is the work of the therapist? What aspects of the client affect the decision making intensity?

CPT® separates out a component on clinical decision making that affects the level, but it also supports best practice in occupational therapy. Best practice in occupational therapy requires clinical reasoning to occur throughout the evaluation process: in decisions about the questions to ask in the occupational profile and history, in the choice of assessments and tests used to measure performance, and in the identification and prioritization of goals and outcomes. The CPT® language allows for consideration of a number of variables in determining a level. Identifying and documenting the complexity of clinical reasoning used at each step of the process will validate the chosen level of evaluation code.

This Table shows the language of the CPT® code specifying what must be considered in identifying a level for this component.

CPT® Code	CPT® Descriptors
Low Complexity (97165)	Clinical decision making of **low complexity**, which includes an analysis of the occupational profile, analysis of data from **problem-focused assessment(s),** and consideration of a **limited number** of treatment options. Patient presents with no comorbidities that affect occupational performance. **Modification** of tasks or assistance (e.g., physical or verbal) with assessment(s) is **not necessary** to enable completion of evaluation component.
Moderate Complexity (97166)	Clinical decision making of **moderate analytic complexity,** which includes an analysis of the occupational profile, analysis of data from **detailed assessment(s),** and consideration of **several treatment options**. Patient may present with comorbidities that affect occupational performance. Minimal to moderate modification of tasks or assistance (e.g., physical or verbal) with assessment(s) is necessary to enable completion of evaluation component.
High Complexity (97167)	Clinical decision making of **high analytic complexity**, which includes an analysis of the occupational profile, analysis of data from **comprehensive assessment(s),** and consideration of **multiple treatment options**. Patient may present with comorbidities that affect occupational performance. **Significant modification** of tasks or assistance (e.g., physical or verbal) with assessment(s) is **necessary to enable patient to complete evaluation component.**

Specified Criteria for Clinical Decision Making Level
The CPT® language provides clear delineation of factors that can be related to not only the determination of the clinical decision making component but also factors that affect other components. The code language speaks to interrelated factors and thus an interrelated process that must be considered in determining the level of clinical decision making.

Assessment Process
As noted in the previous section on assessment and performance deficit identification, this section on clinical decision making describes levels of analysis and assessment that are useful in determining the level of both the assessment and clinical decision-making component. For illustration, this Table is repeated.

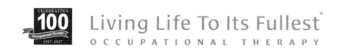

Living Life To Its Fullest®
OCCUPATIONAL THERAPY

4720 Montgomery Lane, Bethesda, MD 20814-3425
Phone: 301-652-2682 TDD: 800-377-8555 Fax: 301-652-7711

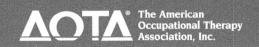

CPT° Code	CPT° Descriptors
Low Complexity (97165)	Analysis of data from problem-focused assessment(s)
Moderate Complexity (97166)	Analysis of data from detailed assessment(s)
High Complexity (97167)	Analysis of data from comprehensive assessment(s)

Comorbidities

The type, number, and complexity of *comorbidities* affecting occupational performance or that result in participation restrictions are identified as affecting the evaluation code level.

Comorbidities are not explicitly defined in the CPT® language but elsewhere are defined as:

> *The presence of one or more additional diseases, conditions, or disorders that are concurrent with a primary disease or disorder and may impact client complexity. Co-morbidities can also include socioeconomic, cultural, environmental, and client behavior characteristics.* (Valderas, Starfield, Sibbald, Salisbury, & Roland, 2009)

For example, a secondary diagnosis of chronic obstructive pulmonary disease (COPD) may influence the client's breathing and fatigue level, affecting completion of desired activities of daily living. Another common comorbidity is problems in cognition; for instance, following an acute hospitalization. Cognitive problems can negatively affect sequencing or other factors necessary to complete activities of daily living.

Assessment Modification and Need for Assistance

When a client has difficulty with an assessment, the therapist may need to make modification of directions, task complexity, environment, time, or other factors. The therapist may need to make such adjustments in the assessment to get a clear picture of the scope of performance deficits resulting in activity limitations and/or performance limitations.

The CPT® language describes the levels of assistance or modification that may be needed to enable completion of assessments that contribute to the level of clinical decision making. The language also gives examples that assistance may be physical, verbal, or some other form. Any modifications or adjustments in assessing performance deficits and activity limitations should be documented to show relationship to the level of evaluation code to choose.

CPT° Code	CPT° Descriptors
Low Complexity (97165)	Modification of tasks or assistance is not necessary
Moderate Complexity (97166)	Minimal to moderate modification of tasks is necessary
High Complexity (97167)	Significant modification of tasks or assistance is necessary

Selection of Interventions

Selecting from multiple options as opposed to considering limited options raises the level of clinical decision making. For instance, treatment of hemiparesis may involve choosing among several options for treatment, adaptation, or compensatory activities. But treatment of a shoulder hemi-arthroplasty may be driven primarily by a limited number of treatment options.

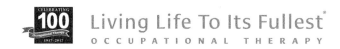

Living Life To Its Fullest
OCCUPATIONAL THERAPY

4720 Montgomery Lane, Bethesda, MD 20814-3425
Phone: 301-652-2682 TDD: 800-377-8555 Fax: 301-652-7711

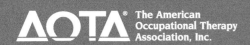

CPT° Code	CPT° Descriptors
Low Complexity (97165)	Consideration of a limited number of treatment options
Moderate Complexity (97166)	Consideration of several treatment options
High Complexity (97167)	Consideration of multiple treatment options

Time

The new evaluation and re-evaluation codes are considered *service codes*; they are not time-based codes. Although the AMA has typical times associated with each of the codes, time is not the determining factor in selection of the code. One unit of an evaluation code is submitted regardless of the amount of time spent on the evaluation; the complexity of the evaluation determines which level of code is selected.

While the code language provides typical times for each of the three levels of evaluation, the time is not an absolute requirement. It is simply a general guideline about how long each of the levels of evaluation codes might take. **Time Cannot Be Used as a Factor in Determining Levels. This is not part of the equation for determination in the CPT process.** Therapists must not be pressured to use time as a critical factor. The previously discussed criteria of history, assessment and deficits, and clinical judgment are the criteria that determine the level. Typical times are included in the following Table simply to reflect that there are differences in time when considering three levels of evaluation.

CPT° Code	Typical Face-to-Face Time
Low Complexity (97165)	30 minutes
Moderate Complexity (97166)	45 minutes
High Complexity (97167)	60 minutes

The typical times identified should not be construed as either requirements or limits. In some ways, the typical times can help to defend the time needed for full and complete evaluations. However, the differences may present scheduling problems. Many of these issues will be addressed as the codes are fully utilized. It is important for therapists to understand what typical times mean and be prepared to defend and document the time they need for any evaluation level.

Plan of Care

The code language references the development of the plan of care as the final step in evaluation. The plan of care is written after all information is gathered and analyzed from the client's history, occupational profile, activity limitation and/or participation restrictions, and standardized and non-standardized assessments. The therapist's clinical reasoning and critical thinking skills provide a meaningful interpretation of the data in order to develop an effective treatment plan. The plan of care identifies the intervention strategies needed to improve the client's functional performance. The plan of care identifies the specialized skills occupational therapy uses to achieve desired outcomes and substantiates the medical necessity of providing occupational therapy. Outcome goals are established to track the progress of intervention and identify occupational therapy's distinct value. The plan of care is reviewed on an ongoing basis throughout the intervention process/episode to assure that therapeutic priorities continue to be met.

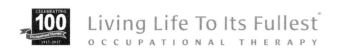

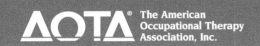

REEVALUATION

Reevaluation: Reappraisal of the client's performance and goals to determine the type and amount of change that has taken place. (AOTA, 2014, p. S45)

While there are no levels of reevaluation, the CPT® language provides similar guidance for the components of the reevaluation. CPT® does not speak to when a reevaluation can take place; those guidelines are usually provided by payers.

CPT° Code Components	CPT° Descriptors
Assessment	An assessment of changes in patient functional or medical status with revised plan of care.
Occupational Profile	An update to the initial occupational profile to reflect changes in condition or environment that affect future interventions and/or goals.
Plan of Care	A revised plan of care. A formal reevaluation is performed when there is a documented change in functional status, or a significant change to the plan of care is required.

Payers such as Medicare and private insurance may have particular rules about when a re-evaluation is reimbursable. The CPT® language only describes the items required to bill the code.

As with the evaluation codes, a typical time is stated as 30 minutes of face-to-face interaction with the patient or family. Again, this is not to be considered a requirement or a limit on time.

Defending Appropriate Levels of Evaluation Codes

As noted earlier in the document, following this approach for conducting an evaluation provides opportunities to practice consistent with the *Framework* as well as in optimal, best practice ways. Approaching evaluation comprehensively will help to promote the distinct value of occupational therapy in the evolving health care system.

The transition to these new codes may be challenging for therapists and administrators. But the codes are clear in their requirements. The components must be identified and justified in the documentation. Therapists must be clear with administrators that evaluation is a process not defined by the same amount of time or level for each client, but rather by the intensity and complexity of the client's individual performance deficits.

Arming oneself with knowledge of the evaluation code components will enable defense of appropriate evaluation code selection in any outside or internal review.

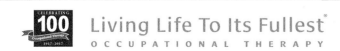

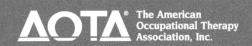

**The American
Occupational Therapy
Association, Inc.**

www.aota.org

New Occupational Therapy Evaluation Coding Overview

SUMMARY

Evaluation Code	Occupational Profile and Medical/Therapy History	Patient Assessment	Clinical Decision Making
Low complexity (97165)	Brief history relating to presenting problem	Problem-focused. 1-3 performance deficits relating to physical, cognitive, psychosocial limitations/restrictions	Low complexity, limited amount of treatment options, no assessment modification, no co-morbidities
Moderate complexity (97166)	Expanded review of therapy/medical records. Additional review of physical, cognitive, psychosocial performance	Detailed. 3-5 performance deficits relating to physical, cognitive, psychosocial limitations/restrictions	Moderate analytical complexity, detailed assessments, minimal to moderate modification of assessments, may have comorbidities.
High complexity (97167)	Extensive review of physical, cognitive, psychosocial performance	Comprehensive, 5 or more performance deficits relating to physical, cognitive, and psychosocial limitations/restrictions.	High analytical complexity, comprehensive assessments, multiple treatment options, significant modifications of assessment, comorbidities affecting performance.

While the move to three levels of evaluation may seem daunting, the language of the CPT® supports a holistic and broad view of an occupational therapy evaluation. This follows the Framework in encompassing the importance of an occupational profile and the analysis of occupational performance. Proper use of the codes and appropriate identification of a level will create data to further show the breadth of occupational therapy practice. While at the time of this writing Medicare may pay the same for each level, other payers may determine different payment for each. Furthermore, as noted earlier, it is ethically and often legally required that the therapist report the correct code for any service provided.

References

American Medical Association (2016). *Current Procedural Terminology: CPT® 2017 professional edition.* Chicago: Author. Current Procedural Terminology is copyright 1966, 1970, 1973, 1977, 1981, 1983–2016 by the American Medical Association. All rights reserved.

American Occupational Therapy Association. (2014). Occupational therapy practice framework: Domain and process (3rd ed.). *American Journal of Occupational Therapy, 68,* S1–S48. http://dx.doi.org/10.5014/ajot.2014.682006

Valderas, J. M., Starfield, B., Sibbald, B., Salisbury, C., & Roland, M. (2009). Defining comorbidity: Implications for understanding health and health services. *Annals of Family Medicine, 7,* 357–363. http://dx.doi.org/10.1370/afm.983

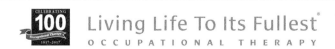